FEATUR

SUMMER 2025 • NUM

PERSONAL HISTORY

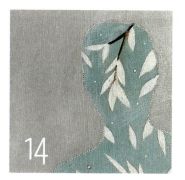

14

Citizen of Two Kingdoms
Aberdeen Livingstone

Living with a chronic illness, I've traveled between the kingdom of health and the kingdom of sickness.

ESSAY

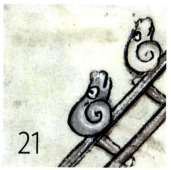

21

Against Optimization
David Zahl

The wellness industry sells you a version of yourself it can't deliver. Hope lies elsewhere.

ESSAY

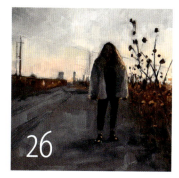

26

Sharon Leaves the House
Abraham M. Nussbaum

My first psychiatric patient taught me the wonder, and the limits, of therapy.

PHOTO ESSAY

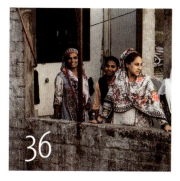

36

Bhopal Today
Cristiano Dennani

Forty years after history's worst industrial disaster, survivors still live in its shadow.

REPORT

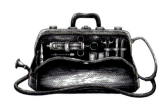

72

A Better Way to Doctor
Brewer Eberly

The direct primary care model aims to put relationships over profit.

ESSAY

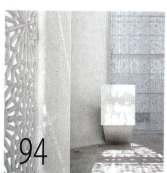

94

Abraham's Warring Children
Kelsey Osgood

After October 7, can a Jewish-Christian-Muslim center in Abu Dhabi make any difference?

Plough

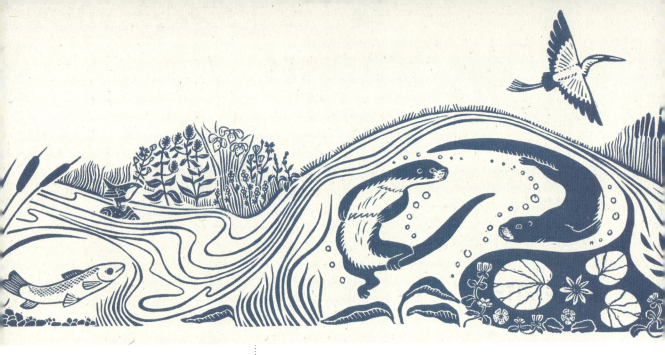

INSIGHTS

FROM THE EDITOR

11 **What Is Health?**
To be healthy is to be whole. That is more than the individualistic pursuit of wellness can provide.
Peter Mommsen

PERSONAL HISTORY

32 **A Disabled Savior**
The wounds of a resurrected God help us live with ours.
Devan Stahl

INTERVIEW

46 **In Pursuit of Homefulness**
Health is not the absence of illness.
John Swinton

ESSAY

50 **In Defense of Pint and Pipe**
Smoking and drinking carry known risks. Here's why I haven't given them up.
Malcolm Guite

REPORT

54 **Of Antarctic Ice and Ocean Currents**
On an icebreaker in the Weddell Sea, I felt a warming planet's pulse.
Jessica T. Miskelly

READINGS

61 **Health Is Belonging**
Edith Stein, Wendell Berry, Teresa of Ávila, Christoph F. Blumhardt

ESSAY

66 **What Families with Autistic Children Know**
For parents of neurodiverse children, church and school can be another hurdle.
Sam Tomlin

PERSONAL HISTORY

82 **Desire, Use, Repeat**
An addict looks for a way out.
James Mumford

DISPATCH

88 **Healing at Annoor**
A hospital in Mafraq, Jordan, serves patients with tuberculosis.
Heather M. Surls

REPORT

101 **Who Cares for the Carers?**
Hidden in plain sight, foreign health aides in UK nursing homes face exploitation.
Hazel Thompson

DEPARTMENTS

LETTERS

4 **Readers Respond**

FAMILY AND FRIENDS

7 **Growing Roots in Portugal**
Claudio Oliver

8 **Orthodox Stonemasonry**
Alan Koppschall

COMMUNITY SNAPSHOT
106 Little Person, Big Welcome
Bringing home a baby on the Bruderhof is no small affair.
Maureen Swinger

FORERUNNERS
117 Bartolomé de las Casas
A slaveholding colonizer becomes a defender of the Indigenous.
Terence Sweeney

ARTS & LETTERS

POETRY
81 On the Staten Island Ferry
93 The Stump
109 It Could Be Worse
A. E. Stallings

REVIEWS
78 What We're Reading
William Thomas Okie on *The Serviceberry*, Coretta Thomson on *Women and the Reformations*, and James Smoker on *The Fox Wife*.

BOOK EXCERPT
110 Armenia's Day of the Dead
Two short stories from *Plough*'s new book *To Go On Living*.
Narine Abgaryan

WEB EXCLUSIVES

Read these articles at *plough.com/web44*.

ESSAY
The Myth of the Nature Cure
Polly Atkin

ESSAY
Food Is Not Magic
Garth Brown

ESSAY
The Vaccine Wars
Brian Volck

Artwork by becca iHorne. Used by permission.

Plough
ANOTHER LIFE IS POSSIBLE

EDITOR: Peter Mommsen
SENIOR EDITORS: Shana Goodwin, Maria Hine, Maureen Swinger, Sam Hine, Susannah Black Roberts
EDITOR-AT-LARGE: Caitrin Keiper
BOOKS AND CULTURE EDITOR: Joy Marie Clarkson
POETRY EDITOR: Jane Clark Scharl
ASSOCIATE EDITORS: Alan Koppschall, Madoc Cairns
CONTRIBUTING EDITORS: Leah Libresco Sargeant, Brandon McGinley, Jake Meador, Santiago Ramos
UK EDITION: Ian Barth
GERMAN EDITION: Katharina Thonhauser
COPY EDITORS: Wilma Mommsen, Priscilla Jensen, Cameron Coombe
DESIGNERS: Rosalind Stevenson, Miriam Burleson
MARKETING DIRECTOR: Tim O'Connell
FOUNDING EDITOR: Eberhard Arnold (1883–1935)

Plough Quarterly No. 44: Why Be Healthy?
Published by Plough Publishing House, ISBN 978-1-63608-171-7
Copyright © 2025 by Plough Publishing House. All rights reserved.

EDITORIAL OFFICE
151 Bowne Drive
Walden, NY 12586
T: 845.572.3455
info@plough.com

United Kingdom
Brightling Road
Robertsbridge
TN32 5DR
T: +44(0)1580.883.344

SUBSCRIBER SERVICES
PO Box 8542
Big Sandy, TX 75755
T: 800.521.8011
subscriptions@plough.com

Australia
4188 Gwydir Highway
Elsmore, NSW
2360 Australia
T: +61(0)2.6723.2213

Plough Quarterly (ISSN 2372-2584) is published quarterly by Plough Publishing House, PO Box 398, Walden, NY 12586.
Individual subscription $36 / £24 / €28 per year.
Subscribers outside of the United States and Canada pay in British pounds or euros.
Periodicals postage paid at Walden, NY 12586 and at additional mailing offices.
POSTMASTER: Send address changes to Plough Quarterly, PO Box 8542, Big Sandy, TX 75755.

Front cover: Tonia Williams, *Blue Eight*, acrylic on paper, 2011. Used by permission.
Inside front cover: Giacomo Balla, *Dynamism of a Dog on a Leash*, oil on canvas, 1912. Public domain.
Back cover: Jet Langeveld, *Lola*, oil painting on linen, 2018. Used by permission.

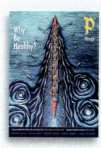

ABOUT THE COVER
Tonia Williams, a New Zealand artist and former world champion rower captures her love for the sport in this dynamic painting, *Blue Eight*.

LETTERS
READERS RESPOND

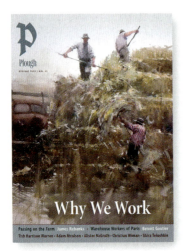

Readers respond to *Plough*'s Spring 2025 issue, *Why We Work*. Send letters to *letters@plough.com*.

WHY CLOISTER?

On Shira Telushkin's "The Improbable Revival of the Cloister": The waste of God's resources in building these monasteries is a downright lack of stewardship to the extent of sin. All the waste is for the fulfillment of a few people. (They could pray as much in their modest civilian homes.)

Do you think a personal relationship with the Savior of the world, Jesus Christ, would have filled their void and broken the chain of humanness within them so that they could have lived a fulfilling life with their family? The answer is yes. Can we humans not realize that radical seclusion in most ways or forms in the present day (however righteous they appear on the outside) is actually self-oriented, which is nothing other than self-worship! Praying is spiritual relationship with God through faith in Jesus (the way). It is not ritualistic praying at certain times or places. Jesus taught that this is the righteousness of the Pharisees and if our righteousness is not better than theirs we will not see God. Would *Plough* quit publishing stories or articles that do not influence people to seek the kingdom of God first, then other things would be added.

Firman Miller, Shreve, Ohio

Is the revival of young women seeking the cloister really improbable? Personally, I find the thought of living as my authentic Christian self while being part of a larger society that rejects and denigrates my ideals much more challenging than the idea of a cloistered life. If we call these novitiates' life-choice "intentional community," would we view their decision differently? People are drawn to communal living for a variety of reasons; these women seek to prioritize their faith. Modern secular society with its techno-wizardry and fake social media has left many people feeling more isolated and adrift than ever. Meanwhile, studies show that people living a communal lifestyle experience deeper social connections and a stronger sense of purpose. These nuns haven't chosen to live in isolation. They've rejected an impersonal society's claims to their time, skills, and resources, and traded them for a like-minded, supportive sisterhood where faith is prioritized. There are physical sacrifices, true, but don't they gain so much more in the liberation of their minds and souls?

DeVonna R. Allison, Ocala, Florida

NOT RADICAL ENOUGH

On Sohrab Ahmari's "The Workers and the Church" (Autumn 2024): One of Ahmari's many controversial claims stands out: his condemnation of "privatism and 'lifestyleism,'" defined as "the dream of a retreat to some boutique redoubt, away from the contaminated world," in which he alleges "traditional and conservative religious communities are drowning."

Ahmari samples a variety of newly potent, anti-modern "lifestyle recommendations" on the Christian right, ranging from homeschooling to hobby farming to investing in cryptocurrency. However, he subverts the trad narrative by tracing those interests to neither timeless wisdom nor the ancient heritage of the church but "the Whiggish self-help ideology that emerged in the mid-nineteenth century."

Readers of *Rebirth of a Nation* and *No Place of Grace*, the left-leaning historian T. J. Jackson Lears's cultural chronicles of the post–Civil War United States, will know what Ahmari is referring to. As Lears recounts, the nineteenth and early twentieth centuries saw a profusion of anti-modern fads among upper-middle-class American urbanites. Trends such as working out, periodically embarking on wilderness retreats, and buying craftsman-made goods all originated in their familiar forms during this period, essentially as means for the bourgeoisie to counteract or escape the negative impacts of industrialization.

Lears appears to sympathize with these trends insofar as they represent a protest against the "evasive banality" and "weightlessness" of a society in which "all that is solid melts into air." Ultimately, though, he condemns them for merely resisting the liberal economic system on liberalism's own terms: those of individualistic consumer choices.

Ahmari's critique of bourgeois anti-modernism in its current, more religiously tinted manifestations falls on very similar lines to this: "There is nothing wrong with and probably much good about weight-lifting or wholesome organic food. . . . But these things do not a Christian politics make. Moreover, the movement as a whole can only deepen the isolation and solipsism typical of the very modernity its advocates deplore."

Ahmari's greatest ire is reserved for the "elite-trad-lifestyle church," a congregation of largely well-to-do Christians who use their resources to cultivate exclusive spiritualities rather than ameliorate the ills of society writ large. This "gated-community" approach to religion, he argues, "represents a profound betrayal of faith's public, social component." For Catholics in particular, he suggests, it represents a betrayal of the church's "character as a mass religion" with what the Roman Magisterium has termed a "preferential option for the poor and vulnerable."

Stern stuff, but there is palpable truth in it. The communities Ahmari lambasts are far from always pernicious, and his portrait of them may be a caricature, but the spirit of Christian privatism does seem to encourage those it animates to ignore or outright repudiate outsiders, whether they be present-day pagans, less fervent believers, or the urban poor.

Nonetheless, if the anti-modernism of the elite-trad-lifestyle church is not anti-modern enough, then neither, one might argue, is Ahmari's proposed alternative to it. The most he appears to put forward in the way of economic reform is advocacy of "a living wage, labor unions, denser social safety nets, and the like," benefits that are presumably to be secured through federal legislation.

This is not exactly a radical proposal. It is frankly just a restatement of the proposal of twentieth-century liberalism. And while it might mitigate some injustices if taken up, even then, it would hardly disrupt the United States' economic system as a whole. *New Polity*'s counsel that Catholics completely cut ties with the stock market is more stridently anti-capitalist than anything Ahmari has proffered.

Pressing for a new New Deal or Great Society regime at the federal level, moreover, is not as much an affirmation of man's social obligations as Ahmari seems to think it is. This is due to a straightforward, albeit often overlooked, problem of scale. Simply put, the average American has little influence over goings-on in Washington, DC.

Indeed, for vast swaths of the country, national politics is actually a distraction from the arena in which people's authentic responsibilities more nearly lie: that of local politics. Perhaps the place most in need of Christians' faithful presence is neither the trad homestead nor the halls of Congress, but the local city hall. Perhaps the venue in which believers should first seek to fulfill their social obligations is neither the boutique parish nor the new-right blogosphere, but the nearest soup kitchen.

Ahmari is correct to point out the pitfalls of privatism, and his pro-worker stance deserves a sound hearing in our national

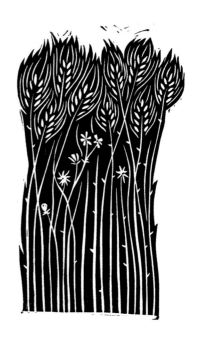

About Us

Plough is published by the Bruderhof, an international community of families and singles seeking to follow Jesus together. Members of the Bruderhof are committed to a way of radical discipleship in the spirit of the Sermon on the Mount. Inspired by the first church in Jerusalem (Acts 2 and 4), they renounce private property and share everything in common in a life of nonviolence, justice, and service to neighbors near and far. There are twenty-nine Bruderhof settlements in both rural and urban locations in the United States, England, Germany, Australia, Paraguay, South Korea, and Austria, with around 3000 people in all. To learn more or arrange a visit, see the community's website at bruderhof.com.

Plough features original stories, ideas, and culture to inspire faith and action. Starting from the conviction that the teachings and example of Jesus can transform and renew our world, we aim to apply them to all aspects of life, seeking common ground with all people of goodwill regardless of creed. The goal of *Plough* is to build a living network of readers, contributors, and practitioners so that, as we read in Hebrews, we may "spur one another on toward love and good deeds."

Plough includes contributions that we believe are worthy of our readers' consideration, whether or not we fully agree with them. Views expressed by contributors are their own and do not necessarily reflect the editorial position of *Plough* or of the Bruderhof communities.

debates over economic policy. But if Catholic social teaching testifies to anything, it is to the fact that nothing should be allowed to obscure that most basic of Christ's political doctrines: to love one's neighbor as oneself.

Collin Slowey, Washington, DC

THE END OF WORK

I have wanted to attend a *Plough* reader meetup for a while now, but I felt apprehensive as I stepped off the metro in Washington, DC, with my magazine under my arm because I hadn't even finished half of the recent issue *Why We Work*. As I explained to some of the wonderful people I met that evening, though I usually read the magazine cover-to-cover within a week of getting it in the mail, I put this issue aside for a month without opening it.

In late January, my wife was laid off from her job staffing and implementing foreign aid projects. My own job with the

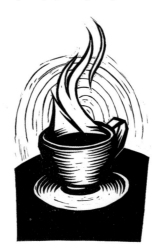

federal government remains at risk. For weeks we each woke up after a few hours of sleep thinking of what we would do if we were both out of work.

In these past months every few weeks has brought changes to our work. As it feels the walls are closing in on me, my mind races to use whatever degrees of freedom I have available to make life "normal" again. I realize, as Tish Harrison Warren writes, that this represents the urge "to use whatever means necessary to avoid the cross."

Drawing on my work, which involves offering protection to those who suffer often brutal violence, I have slowly moved from a place of resistance to, at the best moments, one where I take "solace in the crucifixion," as Stephanie Saldaña writes. Despite my own difficulties, I can still notice and act on the urge of compassion when I see my tired and beleaguered colleagues who have driven two hours to work, and who I know haven't seen their children during waking hours in days. I pray for the grace to love my enemies, though I don't know if I've yet received that grace or accepted it. I do see, though, maybe only really for the first time, that the freedom of the cross makes it possible to love in the face of hatred. I also find solace in the faith that even if my job and our work do not continue in the way I would hope, that our works do follow us in the small acts of compassion for one another and in the lives at whom our work was directed.

N. M., Baltimore, Maryland

FAMILY & FRIENDS
AROUND THE WORLD

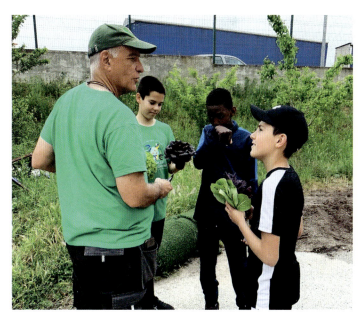

Growing Roots in Portugal

A small intentional community moves continents and finds new neighbors.

Claudio Oliver

After many memorable years in Curitiba, Brazil, our Casa da Videira community (meaning "House of the Vine") decided it was time to "follow the cloud," like the Israelites in the Book of Exodus. This was a moment when we felt called to move forward in faith, trusting in God's direction. Eventually, the cloud led us to Portugal.

In this new setting, we concluded that the fruits of our shared life must extend beyond our internal circle to become a blessing to others. We began to ask what form a community of followers of Jesus should take to embody the good news today, in this place.

How can we be a community in the context of the multifaceted crises of the twenty-first century? Anchored by Jesus' instruction to love our neighbors, we realized that before love can be manifested, the first step is to truly become a neighbor.

Without proximity, love remains an abstract ideal, disconnected from real-world challenges, shared work, and genuine relationships. True love is expressed through committed attitudes and practices directed toward the well-being of others. It is better expressed through verbs: to care, feed, heal, teach, share, restore, accompany, support, visit, dress, and shelter.

Love also involves acts that span generations, leaving a generous and enduring legacy: planting trees, restoring rivers and soil, building lasting structures, researching, writing, cultivating traditions, and working for the common good. If we leave resources and opportunities for descendants we may never know, we also embody love.

Proximity requires careful attention. As Simone Weil said, "Attention, taken to its highest degree, is the same thing as prayer. It presupposes faith and love." In today's world, attention is perhaps the scarcest resource of all. The "attention economy" thrives on scarcity in an era dominated by social media, virtual realities, and ubiquitous screens.

The flood of information and images we encounter daily creates an overwhelming surplus. As with any excess, this fosters a paradoxical sense of scarcity, leading to the overconsumption of shallow content, further dispersed via impulsive shares. These patterns of attention resemble a barely nourishing ration served in a crowded prison.

Such conditions have devastating effects. Homogeneous social bubbles emerge, fostering harmful behaviors. Silos of fake news transform vibrant communities of people into individuals who re-form into amorphous masses, susceptible to manipulation and destructive action.

This misallocation of time and energy prevents the pursuit of concrete, material contributions to the world – contributions that could transform shallow living into abundant life.

Slowly, we are learning to combat the epidemic of inattentiveness using the most effective and simple tool available: paying attention to the people around us. This means listening deeply and acting

---

Claudio Oliver is a pastor and the founder of a Christian community, Casa da Videira. The group has recently relocated from Brazil to a town near Lisbon, Portugal.

Claudio Oliver and some friends in the community's garden.

purposefully on what we hear. When we pay attention with our whole being, we create space for the other. But how?

First, we cannot compare ourselves to others. Comparison centers on us rather than the community we serve. Instead, in our group we choose two other attitudes: admiration and willingness to learn others' rhythms, culture, food, and ways of life. As newcomers, we must take care not to step on the flowers planted by those who came before us.

We must also recognize that we are not bearers of God – he has been present in this place long before us. Our role is not to announce his presence but to discern and follow the signs and paths he has already prepared.

When we first arrived in Portugal, we knew none of our neighbors, and we weren't sure how to connect with new people in a different culture. Having left behind fifty years of networks and connections that provided me with a clear way to navigate life, I was filled with more doubts than certainties.

We had to start somewhere, so we began by transforming our small, bare backyard into an urban garden using pallets, buckets, and flower pots to create raised beds. Soon we had cabbages, tomatoes, strawberries, and beans.

I was disassembling pallets one day when a young neighbor stopped to comment, "Good morning! What you're doing here is really five stars!" That moment was a turning point, encountering a "daughter of peace" who welcomed us into the neighborhood.

We worked to create natural composting with our household organic waste, and soon neighbors noticed how the compost nourished the plants, aided by three chickens that contributed to the cycle of renewal. This small downtown ecosystem turned waste into food and eventually drew people's attention.

The next step was serving. Serving requires arriving without a predefined plan and paying attention to the questions being asked. One opportunity came when a local school with some unused land asked if we could help establish a "regenerative garden." Together, we created a group called "Friends of the Garden," focusing on three types of harvests: friendship, food, and imagination. Neighbors introduced their own friends, so the group grew organically. We were redefining the concept of a "community garden" into "gardening in community," an act of service rather than ownership.

These efforts drew the attention of local authorities, who invited us to spearhead a municipal composting program. Through classes and courses, we met new people and families, strengthening bonds in the city. Our work began gaining recognition, leading to an invitation to write articles about the three harvests and the support movement.

Instead of forming a new organization, we chose to support a local one undergoing restructuring – a group with a longstanding history of love and service. We prioritized collaboration over leadership, creating opportunities like a sewing group that addresses issues of fast fashion, consumerism, and waste by repurposing existing materials into simple, modest clothing.

Now we have many more neighbors to invite to our table. Over meals, they expressed a similar sentiment: "I've been here for over five years, and this is the first time I've been invited to share a table." This reminded us of a simple truth: when we experience abundance, we should not build higher walls but larger tables.

At one such table, a friend from the sewing group voiced concern about an area of the city threatened by gentrification and ecological degradation. Inspired by her passion, we are now organizing a group to try to transform it into a space dedicated to an intergenerational "learning community."

The Bible says in Matthew 6:21, "Wherever your treasure is, there the desires of your heart will also be." If you want to know what someone loves, simply observe what captures their attention. Our neighbors are here; they pass in front of us every day. We only need to pay attention and see them as the ones the Lord asks us to get closer to, become friends with, and love.

Orthodox Stonemasonry

A crew of master builders build houses using old methods.

Alan Koppschall

If you stand in the center of the Pantheon, staring up at the blue Roman sky through the round eye in the ceiling 142 feet above you, it's hard not to feel awe. Two thousand years old, the structure is still as sturdy as the day it was completed. A masterwork of physics and architecture, its dome was the largest in the world for thirteen centuries, measuring 142 feet across. When I lived in Rome, I would often go to the Pantheon and lean against its massive Corinthian columns. There is a calmness you feel, standing in its shadows. Despite the constant bustle of tourists, tour guides shouting out their facts, and Roman seagulls squawking for the next morsel of bread, you can rest easy knowing you stand under a structure that has withstood barbarian invasions, earthquakes, and thousands of years of rain, sun, and wind.

Today, on a cold New Hampshire Sunday in late March, I'm standing under the rafters of another structure that gives off such a sense of stability. It feels almost blasphemous to compare a mere two-story building (with a basement) to the Pantheon, but as the master builder, Patrick Lemmon, would soon point out to me in his lilting South Carolina drawl, there are more than a few similarities. He and his business partner, Seth Haris, and their team are building this house.

Orthodox Masonry, Lemmon's and Haris's business, is a cut above most building contractors. He and his team design and build masonry and timber frame structures. They pride themselves on the beauty of their work and on controlling every process of the construction: from design and groundbreaking to the finish work. Lemmon is no ordinary stonemason. He studied theology and music for four years. Then, after graduating, he took up an apprenticeship with a master mason, learning his craft. Many of the craftsmen who work alongside Lemmon have followed similar trajectories. One studied philosophy; another has a fine arts background. Several of the team have degrees in architecture and three are master carpenters, but none have a merely technical education. They are artisans and artists.

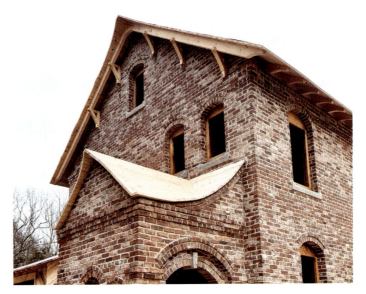

The name Orthodox Masonry is a nod to the book *Orthodoxy*, the seminal work of Lemmon's favorite writer, G. K. Chesterton. As the name suggests, Lemmon and his team use ancient techniques in their building. "But it's not about traditional practices," he stresses. "It's about orthodox practices. We don't want to be stuck in the past using old methods that don't really work. There are true, good, and beautiful methods that have been passed down through the ages that still work. It's those methods that we are trying to put to use." Many buildings these days are built with what he calls disposable construction: vinyl siding, stud walls, and lots of insulation. When they use masonry, it's often a veneer – a brick façade with a non-brick structure behind it. (Veneer-eal disease, Haris jokes.) It's essentially fake, pretending to be something it is not.

"When you're faking something," he explains, "it has to be perfect. Disposable construction has a one-dimensional focus on a particular type of perfection. When you draw a set of lines with a ruler, one wobble is very noticeable, but that's not how true craftsmanship works. That's not how Michelangelo painted." The bricks used in most contemporary buildings have to be without flaws. But when he builds his thick brick walls he can use as many reject bricks as the Old Carolina Brick Company will sell him. Most of the bricks that he uses in the center of the wall had been slated for garden edging before he purchased them at a discount. He recalls the line of the Hallel, "The stone that the builders rejected…" (Ps. 118:22). Because of the old methods that he and his team are using, they not only save on costs but also build in a way that is kinder to the environment. "We didn't set out to build one of the most nontoxic buildings in New England," he half boasts. "But we've managed."

Lemmon doesn't see the path from his education in theology and music to his masonry work as a rupture. Rather, what

---

Alan Koppschall is an editor and an event coordinator at Plough. *He is a member of the Bruderhof and lives at the Fox Hill Bruderhof in Walden, New York.*

The New Hampshire home that Patrick Lemmon and his team are building.

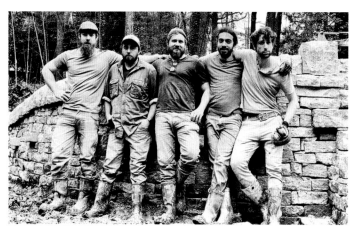

he does now is a continuation of what he learned. His grasp of the language of music has passed over into his understanding of architecture. "Music is a language that is still alive," he explains, "because the people who theorize about it are also the people making music. If I sit down with my guitar, I can come up with a complex chord sequence and work it into a song. Then I can repeat that chord sequence at different points throughout that song. For my architecture work, it's the same. I add one detail here," he points to the arching wooden beam above us; a groove curves along its length. "And then I repeat it here," he points to the fireplace. The same indentation is mirrored in the masonry. "The problem with most architecture is that the architect is not involved in the actual process of building. The language of architecture is dying, but when you're involved in the actual construction of the building, you can work with the materials you have and build in a way that makes sense and is beautiful."

There is a fire crackling in the large stone fireplace in the unenclosed living room. We move closer to it as the New Hampshire wind is biting for a late March morning. The structure of the house is magnificent, the deep earth tones of the bricks contrasting with the large wooden beams. The lintels over the doors and windows arch gracefully. Building with these older methods can add cost and time, but there are some savings. Many of the synthetic materials used in "disposable construction" are made redundant. The thick walls make air conditioning unnecessary and heating efficient, as the house holds its temperature throughout the day. Still, such a house is clearly very expensive. In a housing market where many, if not most, cannot afford to purchase even the smallest of buildings, are they catering to the upper-middle class? Is a home built with this kind of care and beauty only available to the rich? Lemmon hears my questions, but counters. "It's certainly something we think about, but you have to start somewhere, and building with the more disposable methods is not a long-term solution, as the houses will only last a few decades at most."

Lemmon delights in explaining the different styles of laying brick: the English bond, the common bond, the Flemish bond – each has its place. But the most interesting aspect to me is the mortar he uses. Rather than the standard Portland cement, which acts as a vapor barrier, he uses lime mortar, one of the oldest types of mortar. It is able to wick and absorb vapor and moisture, leaving it less affected by seasonal weather changes. It's like skin, he explains. It is even self-healing, the moisture helping to close up cracks and fissures before the cement crumbles. Something like lime mortar – a mixture of limestone and volcanic ash – was used in the construction of the Pantheon, one of the reasons it has lasted so long without crumbling. The setting process for lime mortar is more complicated (it won't set below a certain temperature, so they have to run a heater during the winter months), but done right it results in stronger, longer-lasting brickwork.

In an age that cedes most every decision to the checkbook, building with these old methods is a way of pushing back. It's saying that there are things more important than the profit and loss sheet. "How do you define a good house?" Lemmon asks me. "There are a few factors to consider. But one is certainly this: Will it last for a hundred years and have become more valuable than it was on the day it was finished?" This house likely will.

Poet in This Issue

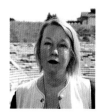

A. E. (Alicia) Stallings grew up in Decatur, Georgia, and studied classics at the University of Georgia and Oxford University. Her poetry collection *Like* (2018) was a finalist for the Pulitzer Prize and her collection *Olives* (2012) was nominated for a National Book Critics Circle Award. Her poems have appeared in *The Best American Poetry* anthologies. Influenced by classical authors, she translated the pseudo-Homeric *The Battle Between the Frogs and the Mice*, and recently published *Frieze Frame*, a book on Elgin, the poets, and the Parthenon. She lives in Athens, Greece, with her husband, and is serving as the Oxford Professor of Poetry. Her poems appear on pages 81, 93, and 109.

Patrick Lemmon (center) with other members of his team in 2022.

FROM THE EDITOR

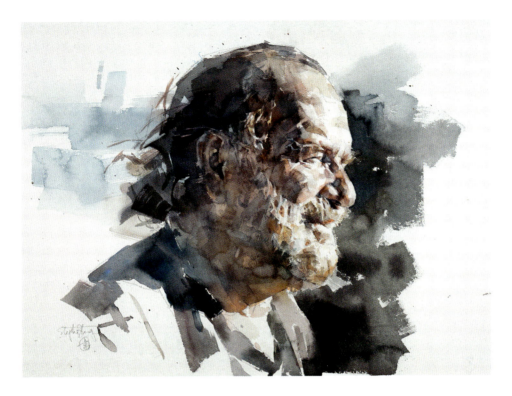

What Is Health?

To be healthy is to be whole. That is more than the individualistic pursuit of wellness can provide.

PETER MOMMSEN

ONE OF MY GRANDFATHER'S best summers was the year he died. Richard Mommsen, my dad's eighty-one-year-old father, learned in May 2002 that he had aggressive terminal cancer. Palliative care was the only realistic option. Shortly after getting the diagnosis, he and Grandma moved into an apartment in my parents' house. Most of us eight siblings were still living at home, and one of my brothers, a nurse, became his companion. Thanks to the steroids he was taking to control symptoms, he felt more energetic than he had for years. Alongside Grampa, all of us embarked on three months of intensive living.

He would rise at four a.m. to go outside to listen to the birds, read, pray, and wait for dawn. When Grandma got up, they would spend time together, usually in silence. After that, his daily social schedule took off. He sat on the patio visiting with passersby, doling out his homemade potato wine (tasting notes: crisp, clean, and floral, like a botanical soju). He wrote dozens of letters and postcards to a lifetime's worth of friends, many going back to the rural cooperative in northeastern Georgia, USA, where he and Grandma had raised my dad in a self-built log cabin. Through the open windows, he broadcast a soundtrack of Brahms,

Stephen Zhang, *Greg*, watercolor on paper, 2020.

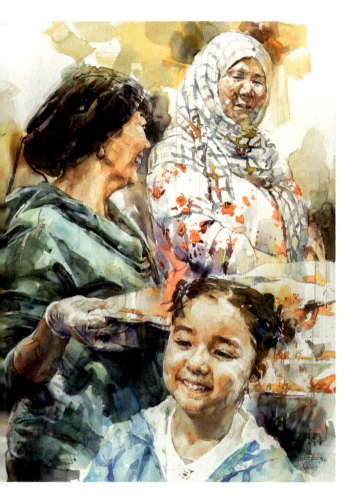

Woodie Guthrie, and Louis Armstrong. In the evenings, he invited his grandchildren and their friends to come over for a campfire and folk singing – the Great American Songbook had been a hallmark of the 1940s communitarian counterculture he and Grandma had been part of.

The summer also became a multi-week literary festival featuring his favorite authors. He recruited us twenty-somethings to read through *Hamlet,* one or two acts per evening. Grandma was Gertrude, and Grampa laughed through the gravediggers' scene as if hearing it for the first time. Other evenings he'd gather the extended family around his bed to read aloud: Tolkien, Damon Runyon, William Saroyan, Che Guevara's *Motorcycle Diaries.* One of his last requests was to read C. S. Lewis's Narnia series together one more time. "Let's have another chapter," he'd keep saying, until we'd read most of a book in a single evening. He'd sleep a few hours, then do it all over again.

He didn't have much pain that we could tell, or any fear of death. A pastor asked if he wanted our church to hold a prayer service for him. "Why would I want that?" he responded. "I've had a wonderful life. I'm only grateful." Another time he told us, "You know, I always prayed to experience just one more summer. And this year that prayer has already been granted." His serenity was in some ways surprising; in earlier years, he'd gone through periods of self-doubt and depression. But now he was simply happy. Dying, he gained a new kind of health.

His "health" obviously wasn't that of a well-functioning body; the cancer's progress was grimly real. Instead, it was the kind of health described as "wholeness" by another of his favorite authors, Wendell Berry. In a 1994 essay "Health Is Membership," Berry points out that the word *health* "comes from the same Indo-European root as 'heal,' 'whole,' and 'holy.' To be healthy is literally to be whole; to heal is to make whole."

That wholeness, for Berry, requires the kind of thick network of relationships that surrounded Grampa. As Berry puts it, "I believe that the community – in the fullest sense: a place and all its creatures – is the smallest unit of health and that to speak of the health of an isolated individual is a contradiction in terms." Here Berry anticipates the findings of happiness researchers such as George Vaillant, who for decades led a Harvard longitudinal study on life outcomes that launched in 1938. Vaillant's 2015 TED Talk summarizing his team's results concluded: "The clearest message that we get from this seventy-five-year study is this: good relationships keep us happier and healthier. Period."

Berry's definition of health as membership in community has clear Christian roots. The Gospels offer numerous stories of Jesus as a miraculous

Stephen Zhang, *Together*, watercolor on paper, 2019.

healer: of lepers, blind people, epileptics, paralytics, the woman with a discharge of blood. As the theologian John Swinton points out (page 46), Jesus' miracles accomplish more than relieving an individual's suffering. They are acts of social salvation. Those who suffer from diseases rendering them ritually impure and socially outcast gain restoration to the community. Some, such as the paralyzed man in chapter 5 of Luke's Gospel, have their sins publicly forgiven. For Jesus, healing is both personal and communal, physical and spiritual.

This background may explain why Berry criticizes modern medicine, even while acknowledging its achievements. Medicine as usually practiced, in his view, attends primarily to the "isolated individual," and so too easily loses sight of health as a communal concern. This isolating tendency springs from its bias for technological solutions. It then treats the body as "a defective or potentially defective machine, singular, solitary, and displaced, without love, solace, or pleasure." Berry protests this approach as untrue to reality: "The machine metaphor works to enforce a division that falsifies the process of healing because it falsifies the nature of the creature needing to be healed. If the body is a machine, then its diseases can be healed by a sort of mechanical tinkering, without reference to anything outside the body itself." But that approach misses an essential truth about what a human body is:

> The body in most ways is not at all like a machine. Like all living creatures and unlike a machine, the body is not formally self-contained; its boundaries and outlines are not so exactly fixed. The body alone is not, properly speaking, a body. Divided from its sources of air, food, drink, clothing, shelter, and companionship, a body is, properly speaking, a cadaver, whereas a machine by itself, shut down or out of fuel, is still a machine. Merely as an organism (leaving aside issues of mind and spirit) the body lives, and moves and has its being, minute by minute, by an inter-involvement with other bodies and other creatures, living and unliving, that is too complex to diagram or describe.

The recent rise of anti-aging medicine offers an extreme example of the "mechanical tinkering" Berry would reject. Well-heeled longevity enthusiasts seek to halt or reverse aging with elaborate regimes of hormone treatment, exotic supplements, and plasma replacement. Whatever the effectiveness of such therapies, they highlight the force of Berry's argument. Can a lifestyle so extravagantly devoted to a personal project of self-engineering be what health looks like? And what about those unable to afford it?

Thinking of health as membership in community promises one great advantage over defining health as individualistic self-optimization: it transcends the physical infirmity that must inevitably find us all. Through building relationships of love with others and with God, health becomes available to those who need it most: for example, those with chronic conditions, those with disabilities, and those who are already old. Or, as in my grandfather's case, those who are dying.

Grampa could still speak and walk until the last day, when, seemingly confused, he asked for help packing for a trip to a nearby mountain. The time had come for the work of dying. It was tough, but he undertook it with apparent calm, in the spirit of a line from George MacDonald he'd often quoted: "I do care to live – tremendously – but I don't mind where. He who made this room so well worth living in, may surely be trusted with the next!"

Lifelong communitarian that he was, he spent his final hours surrounded by his community: his wife of five decades, his children and grandchildren, fellow Bruderhof members, friends he'd known since they were young, and young friends newly made. To stretch Berry's point, you could say he died healthy, the manner of his parting his final gift to the community he'd lived for.

This issue of *Plough* aims to show why that's a kind of health worth aspiring to.

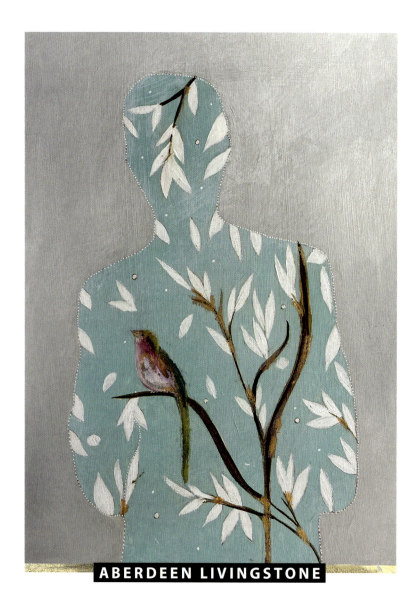

ABERDEEN LIVINGSTONE

Citizen of Two Kingdoms

Living with a chronic illness, I've traveled between the kingdom of health and the kingdom of sickness.

Karenina Fabrizzi, *Maximilian*, oil on paper, acrylic, ink, oil pastel and gold leaf, 2022.

It was in Suleika Jaouad's searing account of her battle with leukemia that I first encountered Susan Sontag's words on health and sickness: "Everyone who is born holds dual citizenship, in the kingdom of the well and in the kingdom of the sick. Although we all prefer to use only the good passport, sooner or later each of us is obliged, at least for a spell, to identify ourselves as citizens of that other place." Jaouad was in her twenties, and fought through four years of chemotherapy and bone marrow transplants before reaching remission and asking herself that unexpected question, "How do I live again?" The title of her book is, aptly enough, *Between Two Kingdoms*.

I had always been more comfortable in my mind than in my body, but in high school I finally found a way to connect to my physicality via the popular and slightly insane world of CrossFit. At the gym, I explored and enjoyed the variety of the workouts, always different enough to keep things interesting. For the first time, I liked how it felt to be in my body. I remember running up a hill and feeling my muscles' strength, knowing I was nowhere near exhaustion.

However, as with others who jumped into the CrossFit craze, somewhere along the way I pushed myself too hard. I began to experience tendonitis in my left arm. I laid off, rested, came back

---

"Everyone who is born holds dual citizenship, in the kingdom of the well and in the kingdom of the sick. Although we all prefer to use only the good passport, sooner or later each of us is obliged, at least for a spell, to identify ourselves as citizens of that other place." —Susan Sontag

---

Her story has stayed with me since, but it was Sontag's depiction of one of the most fundamental human dichotomies that continued to resonate most. I have not experienced a face-off with a potentially terminal illness such as leukemia. My hardest journey has been the quest for diagnosis, the search for some key to unlock a treatment for persistent pain. As I mapped her words over my own experience with chronic illness, I began to wonder if there was another way to understand this dual citizenship she claims we hold.

carefully, but by my senior year of high school, it returned with an inexplicable vengeance. Suddenly both arms screamed with a combination of fiery tendon inflammation and icy nerve pain, from the base of my skull down into my fingertips. I radically reduced my workouts, but instead of abating as it had previously, it grew worse. Soon I wasn't able to type without extreme pain. I could rate a day's direness by how much it hurt to pick up my toothbrush in the morning. Somehow, I staggered across the finish line of high school, a

---

Aberdeen Livingstone lives in Brooklyn, New York, and works in nonprofit development. She has poetry in Ekstasis, Solum Literary Press, *and* Fare Forward, *among others, and recently published her debut poetry collection,* Velocity: Zero. *She writes regularly for her Substack,* Awaken Oh Sleeper.

milestone which now felt like a miracle. I took a deferral from college, and spent two gap years trying to uncover the sources of and solutions to this relentless agony.

In her essay "On Being Ill," Virginia Woolf describes how "the world has changed its shape; the tools of business grown remote; the sounds of festival . . . heard across far fields." I entered into an eerie unreality, as if a veil now hung between me and the world, a world I still inhabited but from some surreal distance. Every little thing became a costly calculation: if I play this card game, my hands will be too sore to chop up veggies for dinner. If I carry this backpack, my neck will not allow me to look at a screen tomorrow. Am I unable to go to college because I spent too long hunched over my phone? Guilt threaded itself into every sensation of pain. If only I had had more restraint, stayed more still, did even less . . .

It has been eight years. In some ways not much has changed, and everything has changed. I improved after the first few years, and then plateaued at what I have been forced to admit is my new normal. I have learned to adapt, to manage. I use dictation software, an ergonomic mouse, ice packs, stretching, all the little concessions one has to make when pain is a threat with every movement. By God's grace and disability accommodations, I graduated from college. By God's grace and a supportive organization, I work a full-time job. By God's grace and the most wonderful of friends, I make it through the daily chores necessary for an independent life.

I have had all the nerve tests, blood tests, mobility tests; meetings with arm specialists, hand specialists, neck specialists, chiropractors, physical therapists, sports medicine experts, and acupuncturists. I've been told that all I need to do is build up some muscle, or that they can't help me unless the pain gets worse. Doctors have suggested a host of diagnoses including thoracic outlet syndrome, but diagnostic tests have been inconclusive. The pain ebbs and flows like the tides, except there is no regular chart to plan around.

Now I live in a sort of in-between. I function well enough that it surprises people when I have to say, "I'm sorry, I can't do that," or, "Actually, I have this thing . . ." From my Instagram stories and morning routine, it seems I am living an uninhibited, "normal" life. The surprise I still feel at this impression is proof that it is not the case.

My not-wellness is more obvious other times, like when my gallant friends carry my backpack, when I turn down invitations to co-work in a coffee shop because I don't want to dictate my thoughts for all to hear, or when I look at the mothers in my church and wonder how I will ever hold a child on my hip. I feel like those blurred glass windows in bathrooms: still technically a window, letting light in but not clarity of image, warped a little, defined more by what makes it peculiar than where it fits the norm.

It is in this strange uncertainty, both of the practicalities of each day and of how to describe myself, that I have come to think of Susan Sontag's kingdoms in a different way.

Sontag imagines the kingdom of sickness as a place where "each of us is *obliged*, at least for a spell, to identify ourselves as citizens," (emphasis mine). It is a passive, powerless thing to hand in your passport there, as if we are Gallic captives being trundled into Rome against our will. Illness of any kind is often an ambush that strips us of agency, viscerally violating our desires and decisions. No one makes plans to vacation in that kingdom. Healing, ideally, restores us to our preferred homeland, where we hope to harbor for as long as we are allowed.

But what happens when you are not healed, when your pain is not fixed with a surgery or a pill or time? Maybe that's the backache that never goes away, the mental health diagnosis that makes every day a battle, the autoimmune disease that confines you to your bed – or even the ailment that has been improved by the surgery, the pills, the

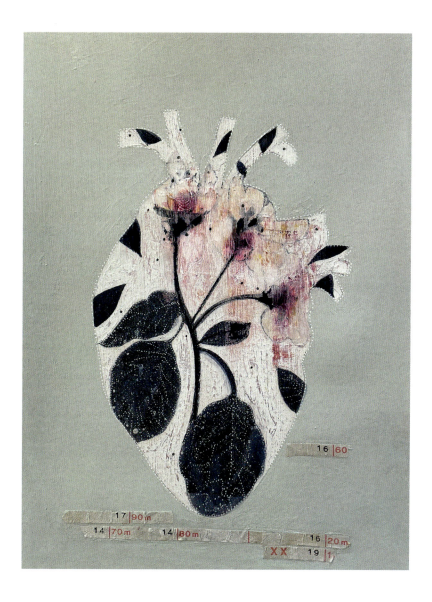

years, but still flares up to remind you that you are not fully whole. In what kingdom are you then?

Some might assume this means you are simply and sadly a citizen of the kingdom of sickness forever, a permanent expat. But for those who have lived with the ups and downs of a chronic condition, the unpredictable swings, the experience is more akin to forever making a border crossing and less like claiming stable citizenship. What if there's another way to see these kingdoms, a way that helps explain and hopefully provide relief for these less easily categorized conditions? I propose we see them not as static states of being – either you are healthy or you are sick – but rather as guidebooks, mindsets, lenses with which to see the world. The constitution, laws, and social customs of the kingdom of the healthy are different from the constitution and customs of the kingdom of the sick, and sometimes, regardless of where we would graph our well-being on a chart, we need to consciously pick which kingdom's laws should guide our actions.

Karenina Fabrizzi, *Heart*, oil on paper, acrylic, ink, oil pastel and gold leaf, 2021.

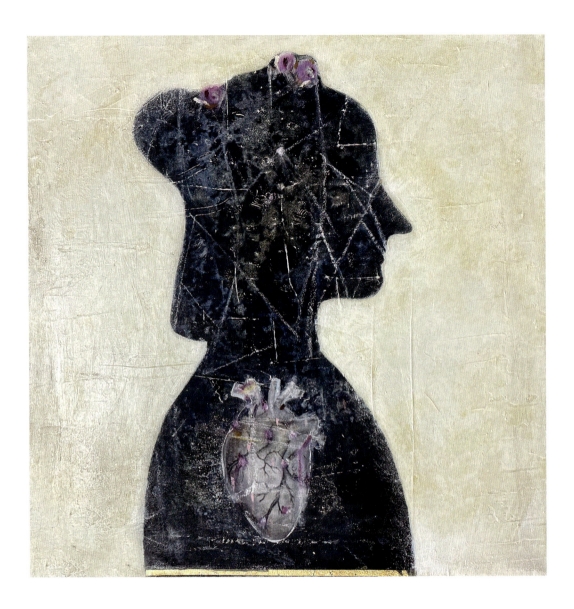

FIRST THERE IS THE KINGDOM of health. The kingdom of root causes, experimental treatments. On the streets, the mood is: *Absolutely not, we will not give in, what can we do to change this?* Its industry is problem-solving, and its weapon is perseverance. Its inhabitants are keen-eyed in their search for what is wrong and unwavering in their quest to make it right. They stretch out their hands to take hold of the next promise of hope, no matter how many have failed before. Their anthem is: Keep trying. It can get better.

Then there is the kingdom of sickness. The kingdom that confines you to bed, or to hospice care. In this land, you hear people say, *This is what it is, what can we do to make it bearable?* Its economy is built on acceptance, and its tool of choice is gratitude. Its inhabitants focus on what is already going right, picking out the treasure amidst the trash. They rest, and recount all the unexpected blessings to be gained in the realm of

Karenina Fabrizzi, *From Fear to Love / Heart 01*, oil on canvas, acrylic, ink, oil pastel and gold leaf, 2022.

imperfection. Their anthem is: There is already goodness here. Keep looking.

The most important thing, the most hopeful thing, about these kingdoms, seen this way, is that they offer us a choice: Which kingdom will I inhabit today? As with any culture shock, it takes time and effort to adapt one's mind to the distinct perspective of each kingdom, but intentional border crossings are possible. When I step into the other kingdom, the world inverts, like an hourglass flipping. Things grate, then fall into place. Suddenly there is a new way to think, to see, to be. It is the difference between making a to-do list and making a thank-you list. They require very different mental states and catalyze different emotions, but both are needed.

Here is what citizenship in these two kingdoms has looked like for me:

Last summer, I was operating in the kingdom of sickness, focused on what I could do, not what I couldn't. I was in the "managing" phase of my chronic pain. I had figured out these techniques to get me through college, and I was using them at work. When people asked me how I was doing, I said that I was so thankful that I could handle work, that it was a gift beyond what I'd hoped for.

That was true, and good. The gratitude kept me going when the pain would flare up frighteningly, or when I was discouraged that I couldn't carry groceries, or type on my computer, or sleep for more than an hour without being wakened by discomfort. But as fall approached, I started to feel stagnant, restless, ready to do more than just get by. I knew it might be time to go back to the kingdom of health. I had good insurance through work, a stable job and friend group, and emotional energy to spend on getting answers.

Mentally I packed my bags and stepped back into the kingdom of health. I made an appointment with my primary care doctor, explained the saga, and dutifully followed up with every specialist she recommended. I went to weekly physical therapy and started researching better desk chairs. I paid more attention to what triggered the pain, forcing myself back into problem-solving mode. How could I make it better? What should I stop or start doing? Just being all right was no longer enough. If it was, I was just wasting my time and money with all these doctors.

I had stepped back into the kingdom of health, not because I was any healthier, but because I was operating and making decisions as if health were the norm, something worth pouring time and energy into achieving.

But sometimes the move goes the other direction. Two summers ago, my pain was flaring up and I couldn't get it to calm down. My family was at the beach for the day, and I sat next to them in a world of my own misery. As I watched all the strong, lithe bodies in the water, I wondered how many minutes of treading water it would take before the pain was so bad that it would impact any later ability to work. I was exhausted from these calculations, the invisible drain of energy too familiar to anyone with a chronic condition. The beach is one of my favorite places in the world, but any joy I normally felt there was quickly seeping away.

Then I had an epiphany: I had overstayed my time in the kingdom of health. For now, there was nothing I could do to fix my situation. Maybe I simply needed to reenter the gates of acceptance.

I remember clearly the mental pivot, as I took a deep breath and looked up at the wide July sky, as blue as hope. I remember finding solace in the sound of the waves, luxuriating in the breeze on my skin. I grabbed a fistful of chips and Oreos, laughing like a kid at the rare freedom of savoring junk food. I made a list in my mind: Thank you that I have such a good family. Thank you that I have the luxury to take a day off work. Thank you for laughter. Thank you that I can see and hear and feel and smell and taste. Thank you that I can walk along the sand. Thank you that I can read. Thank you for whatever minutes I get to spend in the water. They are enough.

And suddenly, they were. Halfway through my mental list, my beach day was transformed. Instead of bitterly reflecting on all I couldn't do, I felt now that everything was a gift, a superfluous blessing that I had missed in my clenched striving to be better, to have no pain, to fix a thing that simply couldn't be fixed, not at that moment.

This time I stepped back into the kingdom of sickness, not because I was any sicker than the moment before, but because I was operating as if sickness were the norm, and therefore not worth my full attention. It was relegated to static, to background noise, freeing up my attention to something other than what was wrong and how to fix it.

Both kingdoms have gifts to offer. Sometimes we need to get off our butts and fight, and keep on fighting. We need to be discontented, to sound the warning: this is not as it should be, and I have the agency to seek a better way.

And sometimes we need to surrender. We need to release our grasp on our ideals, our expectations, our control, so as to see a new way: the goodness that is already here, in the midst of that which we did not ask for. We need to sink into our limits and find a serenity in them that is not accessible when we are constantly on the hunt for better.

Some people claim you cannot grow without suffering. But I have also seen pain break noble spirits. It's not always inversely correlated. Neither is it always in tandem, a one-to-one positive increase in each. But I eschew the x-y axis, the linear graphs. This life is a dance, one foot in and one foot out of these two kingdoms, or else poised perfectly in between, sometimes enjoying a pirouette in one, sometimes hunched over in the other, being spun here and there, never sure where the next measure of music will take you. To stay stuck in either kingdom is not a dance; it is rigor mortis. Gracefulness is the ability to move fluidly, and that, I believe, is what we need: the grace to dance with ease between these two perspectives that together, in a supra-logical, nonlinear, deeply human way move us closer to ultimate wholeness and goodness and glory.

Taking a longer view, we talk of the "now and not yet kingdom," the kingdom that encompasses all other kingdoms, including these societies of sickness and health. We see the "now" when our efforts to find healing are blessedly successful – and we also see it when we experience inexplicable peace in the midst of ongoing pain. And through it all we cling to the "not yet," the promised wholeness that has already planted seeds in our hearts – no more tears, no more pain, rest from the battle – seeds that are waiting to bloom in the final and everlasting dawn. Shalom, wholeness – we are promised this, one day. Referencing our resurrected bodies, Paul affirms, "For we were saved in this hope" (Rom. 8:24).

Until that time, we are graced with tools to endure the "not yets," one of which is this mindset shift that resists long-term citizenship in only one realm when there are gifts in each.

At the end of the day, who of us is ever truly healthy? What is the threshold to claiming wellness? And yet, how helpful is it to only ever identify as sick? What is the line between accepting reality and identifying too strongly with victimhood? Maybe we are all just human, at various stages of brokenness, and the idea of the twin kingdoms of health and sickness can be a guide for navigating those complexities.

What does this all mean for us tomorrow morning when we wake with unresolved pain? In Rilke's words, "Let everything happen to you: beauty and terror." God in his grace has given us many tools to handle this life, and two of these tools are the particular mindsets of these two distinct kingdoms. We each hold a passport to both. When we feel stuck or stagnant, desperate or weary, perhaps it's time to visit the place we left. In the midst of these endless exiles between kingdoms, we need not fear – God is King of both.

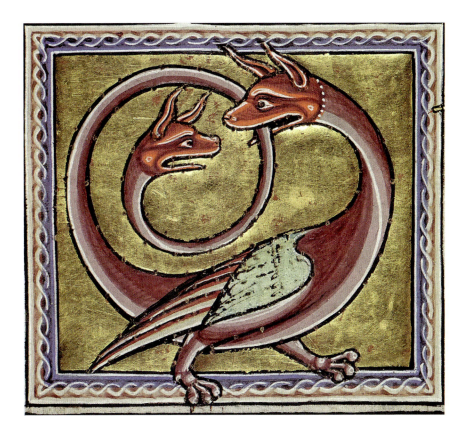

Against Optimization

The wellness industry sells you a version of yourself it can't deliver. Hope lies elsewhere.

DAVID ZAHL

Some people have a gift for polemics. I am not one of them. Two of my personal favorites are Lauren Oyler and Martin Luther. Their takedowns, even when excoriating, are bathed in clarity and passion. But that club is a small one, and even if I possessed the necessary chops – which I do not – I don't think I'd apply for membership. It is too scary a vocation for someone of my disposition. Only an extraordinarily detestable target could lure me into a screed. I would require a topic that not only reeks of malign associations but gets under my skin in a singular way. Something like, say, optimization.

There is a meme that makes the rounds every new school year among parents of elementary-school-aged children. I'm pretty sure it originates from the initial Covid lockdown, but the

Illustration from the *Aberdeen Bestiary*, ca. 1200.

punchline still lands. A middle-aged man stands in a crowd with hands on hips, his facial expression the epitome of Not Amused. Above the picture someone has produced a message from a teacher. "Just log into Zabelzoot, scroll down to the Zork! App, and have the kids work through the assignments sent through Kracklezam."

The meme's staying power lies not so much in its spot-on lampooning of the make-learning-fun website names but in the exasperation of parents at the convoluted processes through which they're expected to guide kids these days. In theory, "Zabelzoot" or its real-life equivalent is supposed to make communication between teachers and students easier. Rather than print out an assignment and hand it to your teacher, you just click to turn it in. And yet I spend as much time troubleshooting the various homework programs on my sons' computers, updating the software, and filling out endless two-factor authentications as I do helping them with their homework. It is a crazy-making experience that leaves everyone frustrated, tired, and not remotely in the mood for learning.

The experience is emblematic of the tyranny of optimization. Peruse the internet or talk to peers at a party, and you'll hear a dozen new ways to consolidate your energy, maximize your efficiency, organize your priorities, and make life more manageable. We are inundated with things that promise to make us, as Daft Punk puts it, better, faster, and stronger.

French sociologist Jacques Ellul uses the term *technique* to describe our obsession with streamlining everything under the sun. In *The Technological Society*, he defines it as "the totality of methods rationally arrived at and having absolute efficiency (for a given stage of development) in every field of human activity." Technique aims to bring efficiency to everything in life. Anytime we use machine logic and apply it to humanity, we are in the realm of technique. For example, we don't refine our morning routine so much as "hack" it. We don't make the most of a vacation; we optimize our time off. Technique is so ingrained in our day-to-day that we hardly notice it. Optimization, I'd suggest, falls under the header of rebranded technique.

There's nothing wrong with conserving our time and resources or with wanting our lives to run more smoothly. What's wrong, Ellul argues, is that technique doesn't accomplish these goals. Technique promises to make life more convenient, affordable, and seamless but in practice makes it more draining, expensive, and complicated. Each new technique we adopt for the sake of greater control creates problems for which we instinctively look for another technique to allay, and so on. If you want to view your child's grade on the homework, you'll need to set up an account with Drumblekick. You get the idea. The first reason I'd be tempted to write my screed against optimization, then, is that it doesn't optimize. Optimization promises to cure headaches, but then it gives them.

I have another, deeper reason optimization almost inspires me to polemics. The lingo of optimization sneaks the idea that we are machines into our common language and self-understanding. This should go without saying but it bears repeating: you and I are human beings, not machines. We are created, not manufactured. We are not "wired" in a certain way. There is no code in our veins. The heart cannot be hacked any more than the mind can be downloaded. These metaphors can be useful, but when we default to them, we risk enshrining productivity as the be all and end all of human existence.

Before long, the same parents fumbling with

David Zahl is the director of Mockingbird Ministries, editor-in-chief of Mockingbird, *and author of several books, most recently* The Big Relief *(Brazos, 2025). He lives with his wife, Cate, and three sons in Charlottesville, Virginia.*

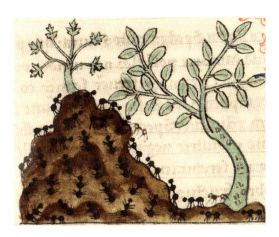

The pattern of the spiritual life, if we take Christ as our model, is not one of nonstop productivity or engagement.

Kracklezam are reluctant to enroll their kids in any afterschool activities that don't produce measurable growth in their child's development. Fun, play, friendships, faith – also known as the most important parts of childhood – these things soon take a back seat to activities that promise a quantifiable outcome. This is all well and good when it comes to machines, which are essentially instrumental; they exist to produce specific outcomes. But when a human being's value is reduced to the output he may or may not produce, dignity is the casualty.

Christians have an added reason to decry this sort of optimization, namely that efficiency is foreign to Jesus. His time management was abysmal; he did not make strategic use of the resources at his disposal. I cannot imagine an individual with a less machine-like *modus operandi*. Jesus took breaks, sometimes at inopportune times. When a storm raged on the Sea of Galilee and his disciples started to panic, Jesus napped in the front of the boat. Jesus never succumbed to the hurry and hard-nosed calculation that characterizes a culture of optimization – sometimes to the detriment of those in need of healing.

Very early in Mark's Gospel, before Jesus has had a chance to do much of anything, he withdraws to a deserted place to pray. Jesus takes a deliberate pause from healing the sick and casting out demons. "In the morning, while it was still very dark, [Jesus] got up and went out to a deserted place, and there he prayed. And Simon and his companions hunted for him. When they found him, they said to him, 'Everyone is searching for you.' He answered, 'Let us go on to the neighboring towns, so that I may proclaim the message there also, for that is what I came out to do'" (Mark 1:35–38). The pattern of the spiritual life, if we take Christ as our model, is not one of nonstop productivity or engagement.

The disciples do not follow their teacher's pattern. Worry prompts them to seek out Jesus the moment he goes missing. They interrupt his prayers, getting in the way of his time with God. "Everyone is searching for you," they say with unintended irony. Jesus does not mirror their anxiety, but neither does he give them a lecture about the perils of optimization. Instead, he responds with patience, kindness, and a renewed focus on preaching the gospel.

BUT THERE IS A FINAL REASON that invites me to write against optimization, the most serious of all. When the "self" prefix gets attached, optimization becomes, to use Pauline language, a "ministry of death" (2 Cor. 3:7). This is a bold but not a hyperbolic claim when you consider the isolation, inequity, and despair that self-optimization generates and perpetuates.

"Self-optimization" has become a go-to euphemism for what used to be known as self-help. The word's evolution foregrounds the perfectionism that was always inherent in more rigorous forms of self-help while deftly leveraging the therapeutic element of self-care, thereby lending the whole operation a moral sheen.

Illustration from *De natura animalium*, ca. 175–235 AD.

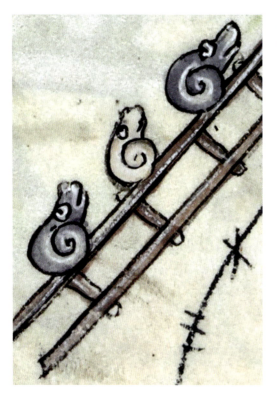

what we need most is connection. It advocates a very narrow form of self-care, which is really not care for oneself (or others) at all. *Vox* reporter Allie Volpe laid out the cycle in vivid terms:

> Companies market skin care products, for example, to prevent the formation of fine lines, supposedly a consequence of a stressful life. Consumers buy the lotions to solve this problem, lather themselves in solitude, and feel at peace for a little while. Once the anxiety, the exhaustion, and the insufficiency creeps in again, as it inevitably does, the routine begins anew. Buy a new eyeshadow, a bullet journal, Botox, a vacation to fill the need for care that never seems to abate.
>
> Because buying things does not solve existential dread, we are then flooded with guilt for being unable to adequately tend to our minds and bodies. We just have to self-care harder, and so the consumerism masquerading as a practice that can fix something broken becomes another rote to-do list item.

According to the school of self-optimization there exists an ideal version of you, and your main assignment in life, as an adult of substance and value, is to enflesh that apparition by whatever means necessary. It is time, in other words, to become the person you were always meant to be, the main difference being that you now have smart-tech to monitor your every step and ensure that you are taking the most well-informed and efficient route to the new you. Self-optimization is a data-driven approach to self-realization.

Self-optimization is almost always a solo act. Nearly everything we do to get our numbers up – of books read, of REM hours slept, of miles run, of meditation minutes logged – involves doing things on our own. The self-absorption isolates us even further from one another at a time when loneliness reigns over every demographic of the population. The church of self-optimization imprisons us in our skull-sized kingdoms when

Self-optimization relies upon and exacerbates the endemic narcissism of our age. Under the auspices of relieving stress, it places a new burden of loneliness on already heavy-laden women and men.

And it places a financial burden on us as well. Self-optimization is *very* big business. At the close of 2024, the wellness industry in the United States was worth north of two trillion dollars. The salvation this industry heralds is available chiefly to those who can afford the products and services on offer, whether those be never-ending weekly therapy sessions, boutique gym memberships, or intravenous cocktails of bespoke vitamins. Modern wellness, as the writer Sophie Gilbert puts it, revolves around "a self-sustaining doom loop of precautionary, aspirational consumption: buy to be better to buy more to be better still." Her description sounds more like a curse than a path to serenity, a treadmill of scrutiny and indulgence that barely masks its capitalistic agenda.

Illustration from *St. Omer Book of Hours*, ca. 1311–1325.

Make no mistake, any gospel available only to the well-heeled and youthful, to those of high energy and/or high net worth, is no good news at all. At least it resides miles away from the gospel of Jesus Christ which seeks the lost, the least, the last. Blessed are the poor in spirit, not the poor in toxins. To write against self-optimization, then, is to write not only against loneliness but against one of the more heartless forms of privilege.

Here the ink in my polemic pen runs dry. I can't help but think that the overwhelming popularity of the push for self-optimization must be understood, at least in part, as a measure of the exhaustion, dissatisfaction, and discouragement many feel today. The embrace of the Thou Shalt Treat Thyself mandate constitutes a cry for help (and relief!) of mammoth proportions. It serves as an indication of the degree to which my neighbors are hurting, worn out, and aware that, as the *Book of Common Prayer* puts it, "there is no health in us." This is something I am not only sympathetic to, but that I feel in my own bones. Speaking of compassion, I do not mean to suggest that all self-care can or should be subsumed under self-optimization. I think for example of the Al-Anon program, the sister organization to Alcoholics Anonymous that stresses the principle of self-care to people who have largely abdicated their sense of who they are to another person's drinking. A far cry from Oura rings and productivity trackers.

But I find one last damning piece of evidence in my case against self-optimization: the despair it instills in those who internalize its goals most deeply. The entire pursuit of optimization implies that our graphs of personal metrics will slope endlessly upward. Therein lies its cruelest delusion. Every one of our life-logging charts will eventually trail off. Age will rob us of our faculties. No matter how many supplements we chug, retreats we attend, or lifestyle coaches we hire, our bodies will break down. Self-optimization is a law without any possible fulfillment, and therefore a recipe for despair. It pits us in a battle against time that no one can win. As a Christian I write against optimization because I write against despair. I aspire to write in defense of hope, and hope does not include delusions about self-salvation.

Thankfully, my faith refuses to let me view optimization as some foreign force that preys upon unsuspecting men and women. Our culture may foster beneficial conditions, but the push toward optimization is so effective, and ironically

---

As a Christian I write against optimization because I write against despair. I aspire to write in defense of hope.

---

enough, efficient, because of the foothold it finds inside every human heart. You and I love optimization because we love the control it promises. What is the allure of measurement if not the allure of personal dominion? That if I can study my data closely enough I can manipulate its direction? Alas, once that line starts heading south, we all know where it ends. It stops in the graveyard.

And yet there are worse places to find oneself than in a cemetery, surrounded by symbols of heavenly rest. Given the fumes of optimization we've been inhaling, we may find that the good news emblazoned on so many tombstones shines much brighter. Who knows, we may come across an epitaph or two that speaks of a God whose specialty lies in the sanctification of unoptimized souls. We may read of a Lord who does not deal with any of us according to our productivity but according to the generosity of grace. We may even overhear words from the burial service about a Father who welcomes into arms of mercy sinners of his own redeeming.

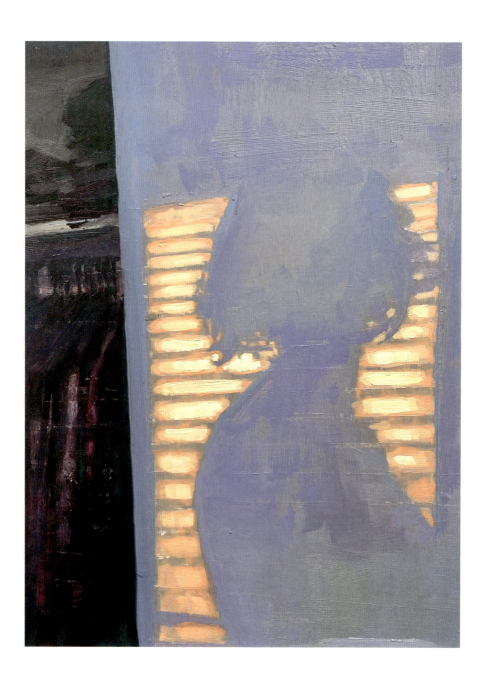

Riley Doyle, *Covid Reflection*, oil on panel, 2022.

Sharon Leaves the House

My first psychiatric patient taught me the wonder, and the limits, of therapy.

ABRAHAM M. NUSSBAUM

"Dr. Gary wrote me a prescription I keep on the door of my Frigidaire: *You must get dressed every day and leave . . .*" Sharon lost the end of the sentence to her tears. As she cried, I silently offered her a tissue. It was the first lesson I learned about therapy from my first patient: you will need tissues.

During psychiatry residency, I learned to carry tissues the way other doctors carry a stethoscope. Everywhere I went, a hospital-issued supply of tissues stayed in the pocket of my white coat. A cardboard box, sealed for sanitation, with a perforated top. As I ducked into some windowless hospital room to sit down in the chair next to a patient on the couch, I would pat the coat to ensure it was in its place. Never for long. A second, a minute, or a half-hour into a therapy session, I would remove the box and punch my thumb down along its perforation to release a supply of single-ply tissues.

There were always tears, but the people I met as patients came to therapy with varied needs. Some needed a listening ear, others a directive word. Over four years, I learned to accompany patients in a variety of theoretical ways – cognitive, behavioral, experiential, psychodynamic – while learning how to listen therapeutically.

Doing so taught me the second lesson: to work with a patient we must form a working alliance. Sometimes people imagine a therapist as a friend who always has their backs, or an advocate hired to pursue their desires. The faculty told me to think of myself as an ally. When I asked how you know someone is ready for therapy, an older faculty member told me a joke: *How many psychiatrists does it take to change a light bulb? One, but the light bulb must want to change.*

Therapists are not friends or advocates, but people who form alliances to help patients make changes they cannot make on their own. Together,

---

Abraham M. Nussbaum, MD, MTS, works as a physician in Denver. A professor of psychiatry at the University of Colorado, he is the author of The Finest Traditions of My Calling *(Yale University, 2016) and* Progress Notes *(Johns Hopkins University, 2024).*

we identify a goal – whether to lift a depression, quit a habit, or grieve a loss – which can feel insurmountable. We develop a set of tasks to advance toward that goal. The tasks can feel clinical – walk daily, pour a glass of water when you want a beer, share a memory of a lost loved one – so we develop an emotional bond that humanizes the relationship by offering an encouraging welcome, a nonjudgmental instruction, or a settling reflection fitting to the clinical moment.

Goal, task, bond. The goal is the why of the therapy, the desired health outcome. The task is the what of therapy, the health-seeking activities. The bond is the how of therapy, the emotional relationship. Therapy works only when this therapeutic alliance forms between patient and clinician. The therapist to stick with is the one with whom you experience an alliance. There's a mystery to why it works, but it's less like making a friend or securing an advocate, and more like working with a teacher or coach. A person who stays in the room, through tears and silences, is one you can trust.

The woman I'm calling Sharon was old enough to be one of my aunts. In her early fifties, she had gray hair styled in a loose bob, which often held her bifocals when she pushed them up so she could dab her eyes. She cried over an unresolved conflict with her sister, over the health of a son addicted to heroin, and over the poor match she had accepted in marriage. She had worked thirty years in a textile mill, moving from the line to the office, but had gone out on disability for breathing problems. When she was hospitalized after a suicide attempt, a faculty member saw her, heard her story, and took out his prescription pad.

Dress every day. Leave the house.

He also wrote a referral to the resident psychiatry clinic. Two weeks later, when I saw Sharon, I confirmed Dr. Gary's diagnosis of major depression and renewed her antidepressant. I told her I would see her back in two months to check on the medication. She fidgeted, then said, "I'm lonely. I don't know if it can be fixed or not. I guess I'll just have to take medications."

I asked why she wanted more than medications.

"God says he won't put more on you than you can bear, but I know you can lose your mind worrying yourself to death. I would like to know how to bear my worries. I can't breathe with all I've had to bear."

We began meeting weekly for psychotherapy in the resident clinic. A couch, a chair, both in neutral colors. An inoffensive landscape on the wall. And, always, tissues.

Some weeks, it was the only place she left the house to visit.

Sharon was experiencing the symptoms of what used to go by the fitting name of melancholia; now we call it a major depressive episode. Medications like the antidepressant Dr. Gary started can reduce or even extinguish those symptoms, but a successful course of therapy can be a way to figure out what the symptoms mean. The kind of meaning depends upon the psychotherapy, but the psychiatrist Jerome Frank discerned that therapies with different explanatory models induce similar outcomes for patients. In his classic *Persuasion and Healing,* Frank concludes that this is because therapies have more in common than what distinguishes them from each other. All successful forms of therapy, Frank finds, identify a socially sanctioned healer (symbolized by the MD behind my name), a demoralized sufferer (the light bulb who wants to change), and a ritualized relationship (we meet only in bland clinic rooms at set times for a psychoanalytic hour). A therapist, Frank writes, must identify a theory ("you struggle to breathe because you feel smothered by unresolved conflict with your father which you unwittingly repeat with your husband"), have appropriate confidence in the theory ("you can get better if we meet weekly for a two-year course of psychotherapy"), stimulate emotions to transform the meaning of a significant event ("after all those tears, you can forgive yourself"), and foster appropriate hope ("you can leave the house, step out into the world, and make new friends").

I saw Sharon for psychotherapy because she wanted to talk about her past and how it affected her present response to stress. Like Sharon, most people begin therapy after identifying a problem in the way they respond to stressful events. All of us experience what Sharon called the worries she had to bear, the burdens and stresses of life. Each of us responds in characteristic ways to these stresses. In a traffic jam, some people offer justifications ("there wouldn't be traffic if other people drove right") or denial ("this can't be happening again"), while others display relationship conflicts ("you always pick the wrong route"), remember previous adverse experiences ("this reminds me of the accident I was in"), or return to unhealthy habits ("I need another cigarette to ride this out").

While any therapy that meets Frank's criteria can be helpful, a cognitive psychotherapist targeting justifications can help identify and correct negative thoughts. When a patient is ready to think about how she repeats the same patterns in relationships, a psychoanalyst can address unconscious conflicts. When a patient wants to overcome past adverse experiences, an experiential therapist can offer exposure therapy or psychodrama. When a patient wants to change habits, a behavioral therapist can change observable behaviors through teaching relaxation training, progressive muscle relaxation, rebreathing, and other behavior modification techniques.

Sharon had suffered many harms in her husband's home and, before that, in her father's home. She told me, "In all my relationships, there was never anything for me. Now when I get something, I hide it." She mentioned the few nice things that came her way: dresses that flattered,

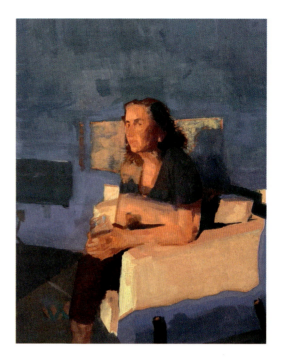

foods that delighted, and our therapy sessions that unburdened her. "I need this time for myself, but if my family knew, they would think I was crazy."

Far from crazy, Sharon needed someone to say what many people in her small town knew but never said to her face. In high school, she met her future husband. She was a student, he was a teacher. When she was pregnant with their second child, he mocked her before the other students only to drive her to their shared home afterward. She never really stepped outside her husband's shadow until she attempted suicide with a handful of medications three decades later.

SHARON TAUGHT ME the third lesson I learned in therapy: there will be secrets. People carry secrets like rocks in their shoes, walking on them until they can no longer endure the feeling. They stop carrying their secrets alone only when they find a place where they can empty the rocks out in front of someone else.

Sharon told me many secrets before finally describing her father. Christmas Eve: a bottle,

Riley Doyle, *Contemplating Light*, oil on panel, 2022.

then another. "He tore down the tree, wrecked the house, and tore up the hardwood floors Mother had waxed for the holidays. Daddy allowed alcohol to mess up Christmas. Mother called her own father. They walked into the woods together. They found a tree. We decorated it and had Christmas Eve in the woods. On Christmas Day, Mother talked to Daddy about the night before. He told her, 'The one who accuses is the guilty one.'" Sharon became the one who carried the guilt forward for decades and into her own family, until she emptied those rocks out at my office.

Week after week, she taught me. The fourth lesson I learned from her is that if you can listen to someone well, she will generally do her part. Over the next two years, Sharon committed to walking daily and leaving the house, first to the mailbox, then to the end of the block, and then to the park. Soon after that, she declared herself ready to leave therapy, telling me, "I'm not putting anything off anymore, not sitting around and waiting to die anymore. I'm gonna live."

Recently, I was thinking about Sharon. I learned more from her therapy than she ever did from me. Deep within a locked cabinet in my office, I still have the lined notebooks from our therapy sessions. I wrote her words down inside quotation marks and fenced my observations behind brackets. Reading them now, I can see how little I knew at the time, how hard it was to understand another person, and how I defended myself intellectually from the mystery of what was happening for Sharon in that room. The only thing I did right was approaching understanding through Sharon's trust.

As I read the notes years later, Sharon now teaches me a fifth lesson of therapy: there will be limits. I was taught to keep boundaries. Never abandon a patient. Never abandon ethical principles. I am grateful for those limits and how they bracketed our relationship to focus on her health. Other limits seem too strict to me today, especially those that caused me to miss the chance Sharon offered to reflect on what God says about what you can bear. Throughout our therapy notes, I recorded Sharon talking about her husband's atheism, her children's wandering faith, and her mother's steadfast belief. Sharon was raised a Baptist but was registered in a local Methodist church. She attended only occasionally, often staying home to watch a televangelist instead. I wish I had helped her experience God's ability to bear our burdens as an active member of her faith community.

Two decades later, after a pandemic of loneliness was declared in 2024 by the US surgeon general, church attendance has declined, and society has become ever more polarized and individualistic, I regret that limit. If a therapist is an ally, coach, or teacher who helps you walk somewhere you cannot imagine having the strength to go, I should have encouraged Sharon to leave her house and head to church, just as Dr. Gary encouraged her to go to therapy. A therapist can offer new ways to think, to behave, to remember, but it's immanent work. At its worst, therapy can make a patient believe she is the protagonist of her life, and the therapist its author. A life is so expansive, no person can be its protagonist. A life is so surprising, no therapist can be its author. Neither patient nor therapist can even be the true narrator of a life. To experience grace and mercy, she needed something more than I could offer. If I saw her today, I would tell her about the limits of therapy.

In *The Theological Imagination*, Judith Wolfe suggests that poetry

> is as important as therapy: it brings to consciousness the work of inhabiting our interpreted world and exercises the skills to perform it. Unlike some forms of therapy, poetry does not do so by trying to eliminate the risk of deception, delusion, and error, because this would be a false

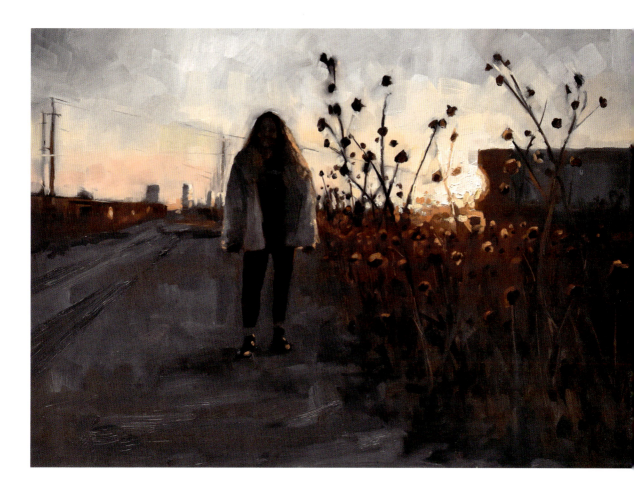

security. We are human; there's no cure for that. Rather, poets . . . tell us that such risk is intrinsic to our lives on earth, where we are never fully or merely at home; and they give us the courage to bear and engage it creatively.

In her way, Wolfe names the limit I wish I had shared with Sharon. There is no cure for being human, not even therapy. Part of why you need to leave the house every day is because we are never fully at home on this earth. Sharon, like me, needed something beyond therapy to fully shift her perception. We all need a mercy beyond the ability of an ally, coach, or teacher, something beyond the limits of our imaginations.

Today I train future psychiatrists. I tell the lightbulb joke as my own when I help a resident identify who should and should not begin therapy. I teach the differences between varieties of psychotherapy, and how to identify treatment goals, set tasks, and build therapeutic bonds. Nowadays, deep down, I realize that the intellectualizations of psychoanalytic theories are there to help me and my trainees remain present in the mystery and ambiguity of how other people experience life. I tell my students that patients come to therapy when the pain is too much to bear, when things are irreconcilable, when they can't leave the house, when they feel trapped by the losses of their lives. I tell them about Sharon. I tell them to ask one good question, then stay silent and listen. I remind them to bring tissues.

Riley Doyle, *Denver Winter*, oil on panel, 2020.

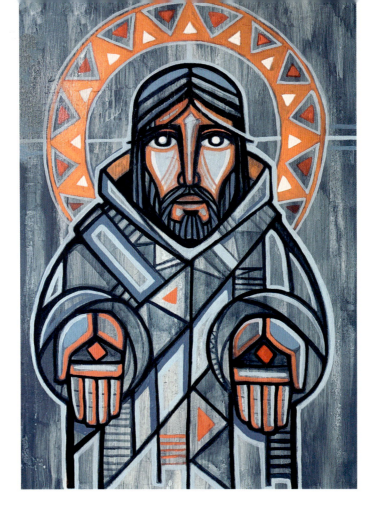

A Disabled Savior

The wounds of a resurrected God help us live with ours.

DEVAN STAHL

In my early twenties, during my first year of divinity school, illness profoundly disrupted my life: I was diagnosed with multiple sclerosis. I struggled with how to cope with this new reality, unable to imagine what my future would hold. I had never considered that I might become disabled, much less how God related to disability. Of course, this was short-sightedness on my own part: while not everyone will experience chronic illness, almost all of us will experience disability if we live long enough. Coming to terms with this reality is essential for all Christians, because we experience God in and through our bodies.

My diagnosis, as well as myriad new medical experiences, led me to pursue a career in theological bioethics. I now split my time between research, teaching, and service to a local hospital as a clinical ethicist. In my clinical work, I spend a lot of time with people who are ill and facing difficult choices in the hospital. I meet with patients and families who are distressed because

Bernardo Ramonfaur, *Don't Be Afraid, It's Me*, acrylic and oil on canvas, 2020.

illness has turned their lives upside down. I meet with physicians, nurses, and other care providers who are experiencing incredible levels of moral distress. Being ill and caring for those who are ill have always been difficult, but the US health care system and health care workers are stretched thinner than ever. As we struggle to cope with this level of collective illness we might ask: Why would God allow this? Why weren't our bodies made more resilient?

There have been times when I have longed for a different body – a body that could keep up with the physical and mental demands of my life. It seems I am never alert, strong, or coordinated enough to meet the demands of my job or to parent my children. It is easy to be disappointed or frustrated when our bodies seem to fail us. As Christians, we may hope that our resurrected bodies will be different. We hope that in the kingdom of God, our society will be perfected and so will our bodies.

Historically, theologians imagined that perfect resurrected bodies would not only be perfectly abled and "blemish free," but would also remain at the perfect age (likely thirty-three years old, the age of Jesus when he died), and some even guessed we might all be thin, tall, male, and bearded (Saint Augustine thought beards made men more handsome). Recently, I came across writings from a twelfth-century Cistercian monk who believed "Ethiopian skin" would turn white in the resurrection. These depictions of "perfect" bodies would offend many people today, but we are likely just as beholden to our contemporary ideas of beautiful, perfect bodies. Many of us long for a body that our culture tells us is valuable. I meet some Christians who long for a young, beautiful, athletic, physically strong body and sharp mind. Movie stars and professional athletes give us visions of so-called bodily perfection that are impossible for most of us to achieve in this life, and so instead, we hope for those bodies in the life to come.

Of course, if Jesus is our example for what our bodies are and should be, then we may be disappointed. Jesus does not inhabit the beautiful, strong, capable body that we desire, despite the numerous paintings and memes of Jesus' toned, CrossFit body you may have seen. What we know of Jesus' resurrected body from the Gospels reveals something altogether unexpected. Before ascending into heaven in his resurrected body, Jesus spent forty days surprising his friends, who do not all immediately recognize him. Mary mistakes Jesus for the gardener when she comes to visit his tomb, only recognizing him when he says her name. The disciples are out fishing, and they do not recognize Jesus on the beach until he instructs them to cast their net on the other side of the boat and they catch more fish. On the road to Emmaus, the disciples are walking with Jesus, and they do not recognize him until he breaks bread with them.

What is perhaps equally striking is that the resurrected Jesus appears wounded. In the Gospel of Luke, Jesus appears to his frightened disciples and invites his followers to touch his hands and feet (Luke 24:39). Here are the places on Jesus' body where he bears the marks of his crucifixion. The Gospel of John describes Thomas doubting the other disciples have seen the resurrected Jesus. Thomas will not believe the other disciples until he sees Jesus for himself and touches the marks left by his crucifixion (John 20:24–25). Caravaggio's 1602 painting, *The Incredulity of Saint Thomas*, displays this memorable scene: Thomas putting his finger inside of Jesus' open yet bloodless wound. Of course, in the Gospel of John, Thomas does not actually need to touch Jesus. Jesus merely needs to point to his wounds and Thomas is convinced. Jesus' wounds are marks of disgrace, of punishment

---

Devan Stahl, an associate professor of bioethics and religion at Baylor University, has written several books on theological bioethics. She cohosts the podcast Bioethics for the People.

and death. And yet Jesus is known to those who loved him by his wounds.

Why does Jesus' glorious, resurrected body have wounds? Why were they not eradicated or fixed or covered over in the resurrection? This is scandalous. It didn't immediately make sense to the first Christians or to the early church fathers who had to account for why the resurrected Jesus did not have a more perfect body. They, too, longed for bodies that were physically perfect. How can we expect to have perfect bodies in the resurrection, if Jesus' own resurrected body appears so *imperfect*?

Jesus anticipates this question. He reminds his disciples that he is fulfilling scripture. "These are my words that I spoke to you while I was still with you – that everything written about me in the Law of Moses, the Prophets, and the Psalms must be fulfilled" (Luke 24:44). The "suffering servant" in Isaiah is typically understood by Christians as anticipating Christ's crucifixion: "He had no form or majesty that we should look at him, nothing in his appearance that we should desire him. He was despised and rejected, a man of suffering and acquainted with infirmity" (Isa. 53:2–3). According to Isaiah, the suffering servant was sent to carry our diseases. He is wounded, afflicted, and upon his broken body we are made whole.

When we long for perfect or perfected bodies, most of us do not imagine bodies that bear wounds. What a strange comfort, to long for a glorious, resurrected body, only to be shown one so marred. We hoped for an Adonis, and we are given a disfigured man. Perhaps we longed for the wrong thing. The bodies we hope for are not the resurrected bodies we receive.

But we should not be surprised. When God's people longed for a mighty, all-powerful warrior God, they received a helpless infant. They wished for a conquering Lord and received a man put to death, unjustly crucified by the state. We hope for mighty resurrected bodies, but we are shown a wounded one. Jesus' resurrected body is not so different from his mortal body. He came into the world vulnerable, and he leaves it bearing the marks of that vulnerability. Ours is not the God of strength and might, but the God of vulnerability, some may even say the God of disability.

Biblical scholar Jeremy Schipper claims that the disability imagery used in Isaiah 53 has been lost in translation. When Isaiah says the suffering servant is stricken, the word used in the Hebrew Bible refers to a disfiguring skin disease; when the suffering servant is referred to as marred and infirm, the Hebrew words chosen usually describe diseased animals unfit for sacrifice. When he is described as silent, this word is associated with being mute, and when Isaiah says the servant is ostracized, he is reflecting the social experience of people with disabilities elsewhere in the Bible. If Jesus is indeed the suffering servant described by Isaiah, the prophets anticipated that he would be disabled.

To call God disabled is likely to offend some people. Our all-powerful, all-knowing God cannot be disabled. If anything, God is super-able. Able to know all, see everyone, create everything. But how can we relate to an all-powerful God who knows nothing of our suffering? The suffering Christ has historically been a comfort to those who suffer. The all-powerful God who created everything from nothing gave up everything to be like you and me. To suffer as we suffer, to die as we will die.

In a time of plague, sickness, and despair, what we need is a suffering God who understands our suffering. A vulnerable God, who takes on our vulnerability and carries it to heaven. The historical Jesus may be gone from our presence, but he has not forgotten or forsaken us.

THE DISABILITY THEOLOGIAN Nancy L. Eiesland struggled for years to feel as though she belonged in the church. Born with a bone disease that caused chronic pain and a mobility impairment, she was used to people telling her that her body was flawed and imperfect. Perhaps she or her parents had sinned, and her disability was the result. Perhaps it was the result of the Fall, of our collective original sin. If she only had enough faith, she would be made well. Perhaps God gave her a disability to build up her character. Perhaps her suffering was virtuous. After all, God never gives us more than we can handle. And if nothing else, her disability would be fixed in the resurrection.

Such platitudes and theodicies did nothing to help Eiesland relate to an all-powerful God. Why were people so willing to connect her body to sin or to virtue? Why had God made her this way? And if, in heaven, her resurrected body was no longer disabled, how would God recognize her? How would she recognize herself?

Then Eiesland had an epiphany: God came to her in a vision, but the God she saw was not the God she expected. God came to her in a sip-and-puff wheelchair, the kind used by quadriplegics that enable them to maneuver by blowing and sucking on a straw-like device. This was not the omnipotent, self-sufficient God she had been told to worship, but neither was this God a pathetic, suffering servant. Instead, she saw the disabled God as a survivor, unpitying and forthright. This was a God that Eiesland could relate to, because this was a God who knew her suffering. The disabled God did not pity her but instead glorified her body.

The resurrected Jesus bears witness to God's promise to be with us, embodied as we are. Eiesland writes, "In presenting his impaired hands and feet to his startled friends, the resurrected Jesus is revealed as the disabled God . . . and the disabled God reveals that full personhood is fully compatible with the experience of disability." In inviting his disciples to touch his hands and side, Jesus overcomes the taboos of disability. His wounds connect his resurrected body to his earthly body and connect him to his friends – we know Jesus by his wounds.

The disabled God was good news to me as well when I first came across Eiesland's book. Like Eiesland, I do not use a sip-and-puff wheelchair, but her vision of a disabled God helped me to see that my own disabilities put me in solidarity with Christ. Eiesland showed me a God who became disabled in the crucifixion and remains disfigured

The resurrected Jesus bears witness to God's promise to be with us, embodied as we are.

in his glorified body. I'm not sure that God caused my disability, but I do know that God is with me, because God understands what it means to live in a fragile, limited body. And I cannot know how my resurrected body will look, but I do know that it will be like Jesus' body.

All our bodies are holy; not in spite of the fact that we are limited and fragile creatures, but because we are. This is how God made us, and this was the body that Christ assumed. It is not always comfortable living in such bodies, in fact, living in a body, any body, is sometimes painful and difficult. But we can take comfort in knowing that Christ knows our pain, because he also lived it. The incarnate, historical Jesus may be gone from our midst, but the body of Christ remains disabled, because there are disabled Christians among us. We are the body of Christ. We who are disabled do not need to overcome our disabilities to be in Christ. Those of you who are not disabled do not need to pray our bodies away. In fact, we enter the body of Christ by breaking him open again and again in the Eucharist. The broken, disabled body of Christ nourishes us, so that we can continue to carry out Christ's ministry. In Christ's broken body, we are made whole.

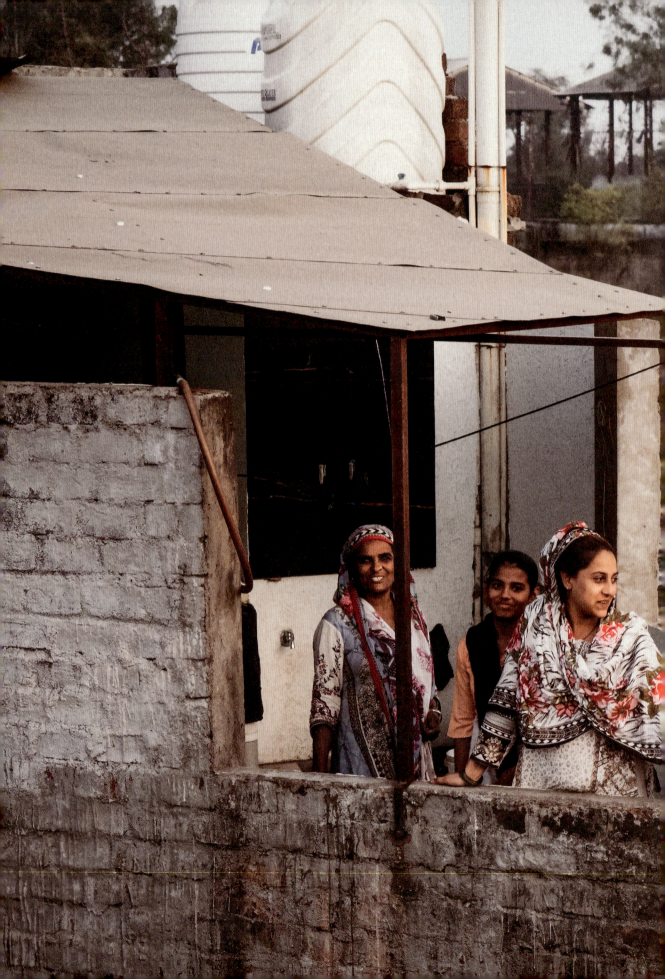

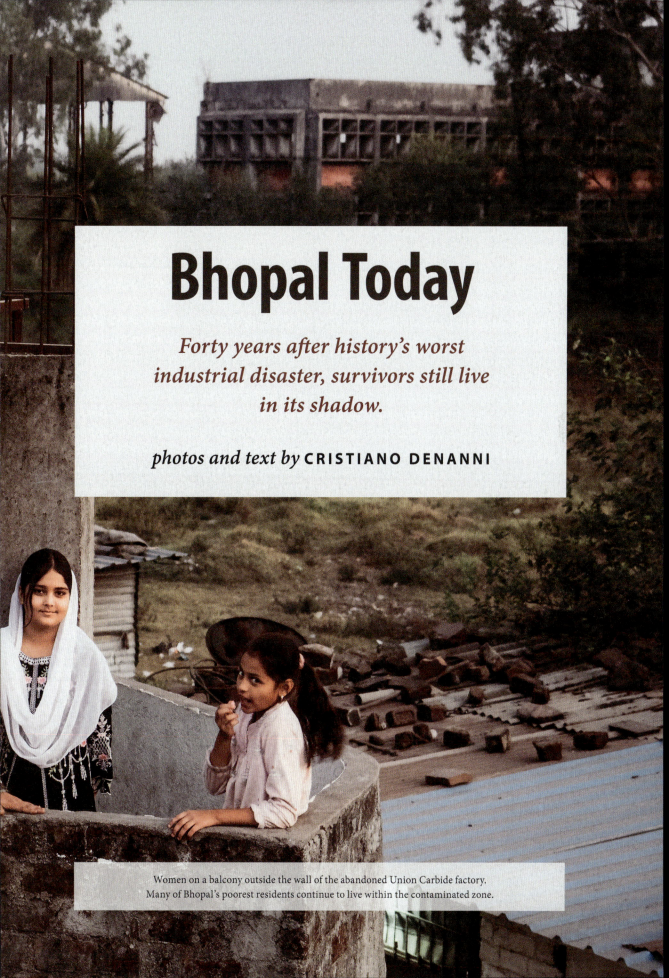

Bhopal Today

Forty years after history's worst industrial disaster, survivors still live in its shadow.

photos and text by **CRISTIANO DENANNI**

Women on a balcony outside the wall of the abandoned Union Carbide factory. Many of Bhopal's poorest residents continue to live within the contaminated zone.

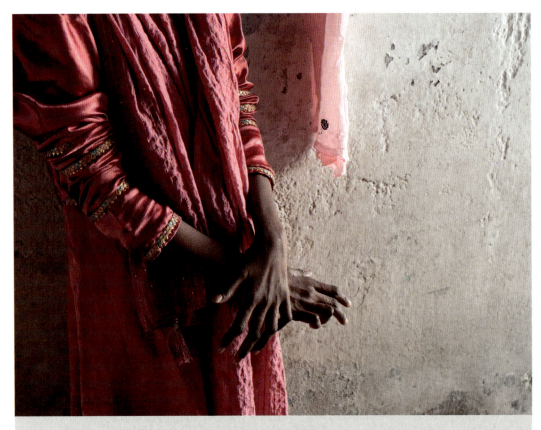

The daughter of a survivor shows her hands, two fingers of which she cannot move.

IT IS ALWAYS THE HANDS that tell what happened here. I quickly learn to observe the speaker's hands. Hands of the sick, of the survivors, of the victims' parents. The hands of a girl unable to move her right ring and pinky fingers because of the effects of contamination. The lifegiving hands of Champa Devi Shukla. As the mouth speaks, the hands narrate, add emphasis, take you back to the origin of the story.

The story is that of the world's deadliest chemical and industrial disaster: the tragedy of Bhopal, in the state of Madhya Pradesh in central India.

In the late 1960s, millions of Indian farmers were in search of an effective yet affordable pesticide. The apparent solution came from the United States. A multinational company called Union Carbide smelled an opportunity, knowing a market as vast as India's could be a gold mine.

Union Carbide had been successfully testing a product that appeared to offer the desired combination of effectiveness and affordability: Sevin, its brand name for the insecticide carbaryl. Union Carbide quickly realized that, given the country's size and sales potential, it would be more logistically and economically sensible to produce Sevin in India rather than exporting it from the United States. Bhopal was selected as the site and a factory was begun in 1969.

Sevin is produced from methyl isocyanate (MIC), a clear, colorless, and highly toxic liquid with a pungent, cabbage-like odor. It is also highly flammable, reactive, and water-soluble. MIC must

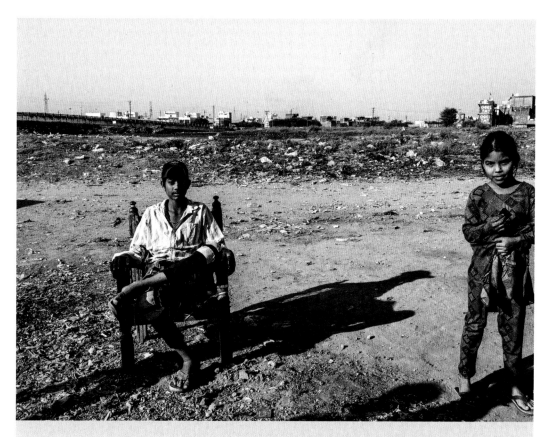
Children play near a contaminated lake.

be handled with the utmost caution and cannot be safely stored without further processing. Even the slightest change in temperature or contact with water can trigger a chemical reaction, causing potentially fatal harm to people and animals.

Even before construction of the factory started, mistakes were made. First, the plant was situated so that in the event of a gas leak, prevailing winds would carry the toxins to a densely populated area – home to Bhopal's poorest residents and many of the plant's workers. That was just the beginning of a series of missteps that steadily compromised the safety of the plant and the entire city; the negligence continued with the deliberate decision to cut costs by skipping essential maintenance.

THE FIRST VICTIM of the plant was Ashraf Khan. As the head of a team working in the department where phosgene – a Sevin component – was produced, Ashraf was tasked with a routine maintenance job on December 23, 1981, asked to replace a faulty flange between two sections of pipe.

Ashraf made two mistakes. The first was failing to wear the heavy rubber gown the regulations required for safety. He was just doing a small,

---

Cristiano Denanni is a freelance reporter and an elementary school teacher in Italy. His photography, articles, and short stories have been published in various Italian magazines.

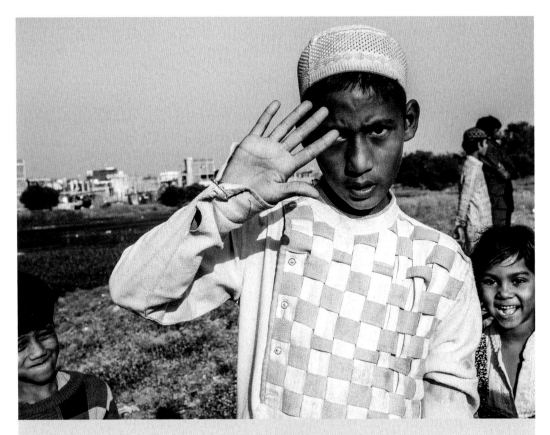

Children in the slums beside the railroad tracks, the poorest area of Bhopal.

easy job, after all. As he reassembled the new part, he noticed a small splash of liquid phosgene on his sweatshirt. Realizing the danger, he rushed to the shower – making his second, and fatal, mistake. Impatient, he removed the gas mask he was wearing before the water jet had completed the decontamination process. The heat from his chest vaporized the phosgene droplets, sending them toward his nostrils. But aside from a slight irritation in his eyes and throat, Ashraf initially experienced no further discomfort.

The first symptom of phosgene poisoning is often a sense of euphoria. That afternoon, Ashraf told his wife, Sajida Bano, and their sons, Arshad and Shouyer, that he wanted to visit the countryside to check out a house they were considering buying. It may have seemed odd to her, but she didn't object. As soon as he stepped outside, he suffered a severe respiratory attack, collapsed, and began vomiting blood. The ambulance rushed him to Hamidia Hospital, a facility funded by Union Carbide, where he was admitted to intensive care. His agony lasted two days. The first victim of a plant "as harmless as a chocolate factory," as an American company executive had described it, died on December 25.

BY 1984, THE PLANT was operating at one quarter of its capacity as widespread crop failures decreased demand for pesticides. As it was no longer profitable, Union Carbide was trying to sell the plant but had not found a buyer.

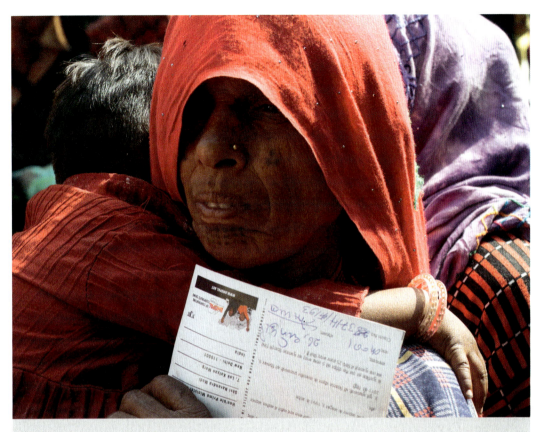
A survivor participates in a march on the fortieth anniversary of the tragedy, December 3, 2024.

As Union Carbide well knew, MIC should not be stored without being processed. This should have been part of any safety protocol. Yet on the night of December 2, 1984, forty tons of MIC were left stored in two tanks. Routine work on some nearby water pipes led to a leak. Since the tanks were improperly sealed due to neglected maintenance, the water made contact with the MIC. Just after midnight, the buildup of toxic gas made one of the tanks burst its safety valve. Within seconds, a poisonous cloud spread across Bhopal. That night alone, at least 2,259 people died, and in the days and weeks that followed an estimated 15,000 to 20,000 more people died, with over 500,000 people seriously sickened.

Many of them continue to suffer today.

As death claimed thousands of lives in the neighborhoods closest to the plant, the deadly cloud spread to Bhopal's railway station a mile away. Eyewitnesses recall harrowing scenes: people in agonizing pain, their eyes bulging from their sockets, contorted by spasms and vomiting; corpses stacked on top of each other; a newborn suckling from the lifeless body of its mother.

In just a few minutes, the Gorakhpur Express would arrive, packed with people traveling to the *Ijtema*, an annual Muslim prayer-gathering taking place in the city. The stationmaster tried to stop the train before it reached the station, where the situation was already beginning to resemble an apocalypse. With three colleagues, he walked out along the tracks, waving flashlights to warn

Summer 2025 41

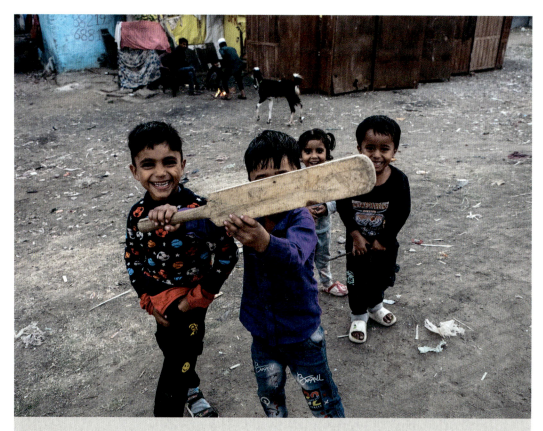

Children living near a contaminated landfill and lake on the outskirts of Bhopal.

the approaching train. The engineer did not see them, and their only remaining option was to warn the conductor – either to prevent the train from stopping or, at the very least, to make it leave immediately, minimizing the number of people exposed to the toxic cloud. These efforts saved hundreds of lives, but many were lost: despite the warning, some passengers, eager to attend the *Ijtema*, disembarked before the train resumed its journey.

In one of those forty-four train cars was Sajida Bano, who had left Bhopal after her husband's death and was returning to settle some family matters. Upon arriving at the station, she quickly realized the gravity of the situation. She left her two children for a few minutes to call an ambulance. When she returned, unsuccessful, she saw that while the younger child, Shouyer, still clutched a soft toy in his weak hands, her older son, Arshad, had blood clumps forming a red ring around his mouth. He was no longer breathing. Within three years, Union Carbide had taken both her husband and her son.

NONE OF UNION CARBIDE'S US executives ever faced trial, though in 2010 some executives of its Indian subsidiary were convicted of negligence. In 1989, an agreement between the US and Indian governments resulted in meager compensation: approximately $500 per person affected. When it was pointed out that the compensation was grossly disproportionate to the severity of the

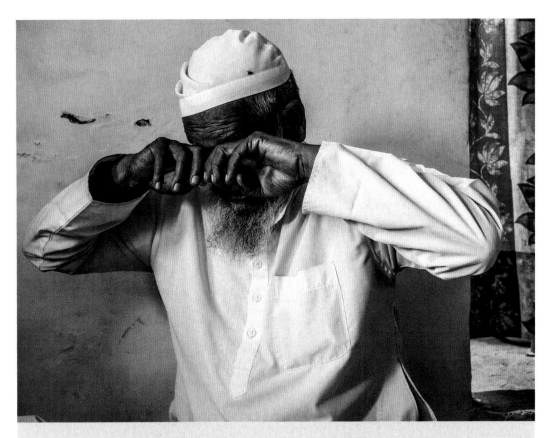

Mohammad Shafique, a survivor, weeps while telling his story.

Bhopal disaster, a spokesman for Dow Chemical, which had since acquired Union Carbide, responded: "$500 is plenty good for an Indian."

In a 2024 report titled "Bhopal: 40 Years of Injustice," Amnesty International alleges that Dow Chemical, in collaboration with both US and Indian authorities, has created a "sacrifice zone" in the area, where over half a million people, across generations, continue to suffer. "Sacrifice zones" are areas marked by catastrophic and lasting health damage to marginalized communities, resulting from pollution caused by corporate activities. Neither Union Carbide nor Dow Chemical has ever committed to assessing the extent of the contamination or properly decontaminating the water and land surrounding the factory, where thousands of people continue to live. In short, Dow Chemical continued to follow the same path as Union Carbide, denying responsibility toward the victims and the environment.

MOHAMMAD SHAFIQUE, A SURVIVOR, recounts the hardships of the years that followed the disaster. He keeps a plastic box of medications beside him on the floor. Next to it, there's a glass and a tablet waiting to be taken. His hands flip through a newspaper from a few years ago, pointing to photographs from the Bhopal disaster report. Then the story overwhelms him, and his hands press against his eyes – tight, rigid, a mask that separates him from a world that has brutally scarred him. Perhaps, every now and then, he feels

Summer 2025

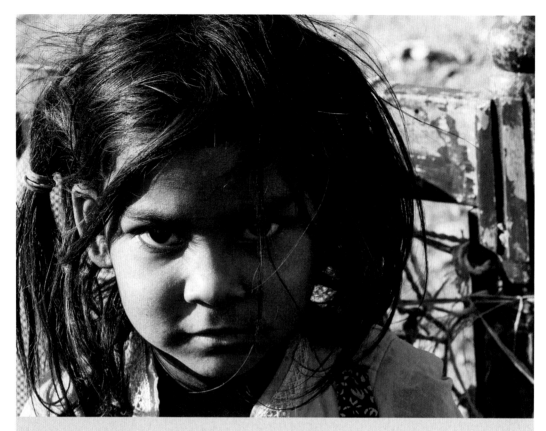
A child living on the outskirts of Bhopal.

the need to distance himself, keeping a part of himself away from his own life.

When I speak with Chote Khan, another survivor, the entire family gathers around us. The room is full and more people peer in through the door.

Khan's home, like others I've visited, lies just beyond the railway track that runs along the factory's perimeter wall, about a hundred yards from a contaminated lake and a landfill. It is an area immersed in toxins left behind by those responsible for the apocalypse, with no effort made to clean up the devastation. Incredibly, despite everything, it is welcoming and vibrant. Sunlight filters through the doors, settling gently on the carpets, and every object seems to belong. It's easy to feel at home in this house.

Looking Bhopal's survivors in the eye reveals the weight of their history and their unwavering determination for justice, but also their humanity – genuine smiles, a desire to share, to rise above, sometimes timidly, other times with unyielding persistence.

At one point, Khan calls over one of his daughters, who is preparing chai for everyone. He asks her to show me the last two fingers of her right hand, bent and clenched. She can't move them. It's one of the consequences of the contamination, he says, though it's not clear if he means directly

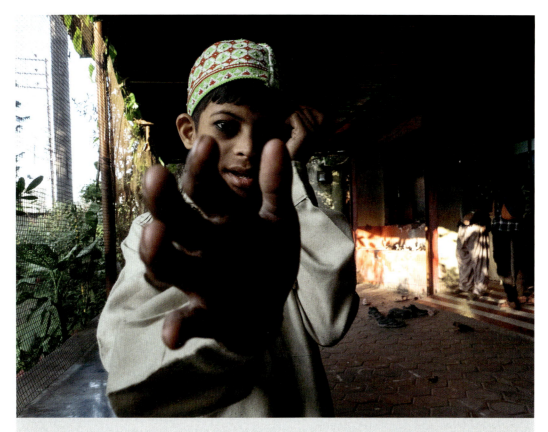
A child with disabilities likely due to parental contamination receives free care at the Chingari Trust Clinic.

or that she was born this way as a result. I don't probe. After the interview, in the hallway, the daughter, a woman of striking beauty, lets me photograph her hands. As she crosses them for the photograph, they begin to tremble.

It's a human reaction, endearing. What lies behind it I can't fully understand. It's as if she's silently saying, "This is my life, my pain. Who are you, and what will you do with it?" The body speaks a language deeper than words can convey. The hands do not lie.

Champa Devi Shukla is the cofounder of the Chingari Trust Clinic in Bhopal, a children's rehabilitation center where professionals from various fields collaborate to support children with psychological and physical challenges or disabilities caused by the methyl isocyanate contamination in the city's soil and water.

I talk with Shukla as we walk through the clinic's corridors and gardens, meeting some of the children she cares for. She's calm as she speaks, a sweet, delicate, wise woman. Her work, she tells me, is a form of resistance and struggle.

There are many ways to resist, after all. Sometimes simply by persisting, like all the people I've met here. Because you can't resist unless you exist. You resist by carrying on despite sickness and deformities, standing against giants without dignity with nothing but your own. Pudias sequi quasperum et as mi, optaect oreprorem in

Summer 2025

INTERVIEW

In Pursuit of Homefulness

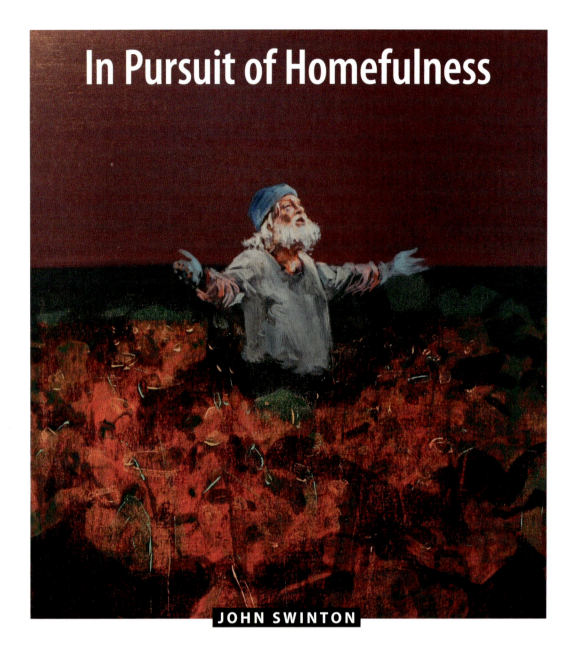

JOHN SWINTON

John Swinton worked for over a decade as a mental health nurse, and was a mental health chaplain for several years, serving people with severe mental health challenges who were moving from the hospital into the community. He is chair in divinity and religious studies at the University of Aberdeen in Scotland, and has published widely on topics of mental health, disability, and pastoral care. In this interview, Plough's *Joy Clarkson speaks with Swinton about how the Bible can help us understand health.*

Plough: How does health show up as a theme specifically in Jesus' ministry, and how do we think about that from a theological point of view?

Bartholomew Beal, *No More than This*, oil on canvas, 2013.

John Swinton: The first thing we need to notice is that health, as we understand it today in a kind of biomedical context, hadn't been invented in second-century Mediterranean culture. At least in the West, we tend to frame health in terms of the absence of illness. With this way of thinking about health, if something goes wrong, we go to a doctor or a psychiatrist so they can identify what the broken part is, whether it's a tumor in your lung or some kind of mental health challenge. You get a diagnosis and then you get treatment from health care professionals, which helps you to overcome that.

But the biblical understanding of health is quite different. In fact, there's no equivalent word for the biomedical understanding of health. The closest term I can think of is *shalom*, which means peace. But it's a big peace. It's peace with God, peace within yourself, peace between ourselves, and peace with creation. There are theological, social, and ecological dimensions to that understanding of health.

The key thing about this understanding is that health is not defined by the absence of illness but by the presence of God. You are healthy when you dwell in God's presence. You are healthy when you live in alignment with how you were created to be. And that does not always mean the removal of suffering or the healing of disease. Some illnesses will remain. Some wounds will not heal. But that does not exile us from peace. Chronic or enduring illness does not place us outside the realm of health, because health, in the biblical imagination, is not the same as cure. It is about wholeness in the midst of brokenness. It is about living within shalom – a space where the pain is real, but so is the presence of God. In that space, health is not the triumph of the body, but the nearness of the Spirit.

The implication of this way of thinking is that healing also isn't the opposite of illness. Healing in this biblical model becomes a way of connecting with God, with other people. Not necessarily getting rid of your ailment – that would be cure – but actually living in *shalom* in the present no matter what your state is. So that tension between *healing* and *curing* is actually very important because we oftentimes assume that healing necessitates curing, but the two are not necessarily the same thing.

We see this in the Gospels – take the woman with the discharge of blood in Luke 8:43–48. Her condition renders her ritually impure, socially isolated, and theologically marginalized. She lives as a nonperson – untouchable, unseen, cut off from her community and, by extension,

Health is not the triumph of the body, but the nearness of the Spirit.

from the presence of God. When she reaches out and touches the hem of Jesus' robe, the flow of blood stops. She is cured. But the story doesn't end there – because cure is not the same as healing. Jesus halts, looks for her, and insists on encounter. And when she comes forward, trembling, he listens. He speaks. And he names her: *daughter*. It's a stunning reversal – from exclusion to belonging, from silence to speech, from marginalization to kinship. And only then does he say, "Your faith has healed you." Healing here is not merely the cessation of symptoms; it is the restoration of personhood. She is healed not when the bleeding stops, but when she is seen, spoken to, and drawn back into communion – with Christ and with her community. This is a radically different vision of health: one grounded not in bodily perfection, but in relational presence, recognition, and the reconstitution of the self in the gaze of grace.

That aspect of healing is so important because one of the greatest griefs of ill health is how it isolates us and can separate us from community with others.

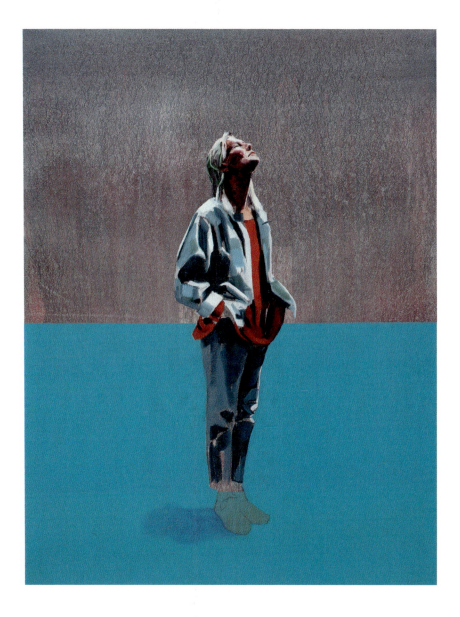

When you have a diagnosis, it can take on the whole of your identity. For the woman in the story, her discharge of blood defined who she was and what her place within society was. And diagnoses often can have the same effect today. But Jesus calls her daughter. It's such a subtle but profound thing to do. And the equivalent of that in terms of mental health would be you'd give people back their names. You don't think about schizophrenics or depressives, you think about people. And even physical illnesses are the same because a lot of physical illnesses are quite stigmatized in that way. There's something very powerful in that dynamic of giving people back their names, respecting them for who they are, rather than allowing whatever condition they're living with to overtake the whole of who they are.

Bartholomew Beal, *Neither Here nor There*, oil on canvas, 2017.

When I was in grad school we discussed a painting depicting the resurrection of the dead. The artist had painted what he thought would be resurrection bodies: healthy, flawless thirty-three-year-old bodies, the age that Jesus was resurrected. While most of us would reject the idea that Kim Kardashian is more spiritual than a normal person by virtue of her perfect body, it does bring up an interesting question: How do we think about resurrected bodies and imperfections?

When it comes to heavenly things, the first thing to notice is that the Bible doesn't give us very much information. We're constantly projecting onto our ideas of heaven and resurrection bodies from where we are. And who tells you what is beautiful? The media. You look at images on the internet or in magazines and you think, oh, that's beautiful, that's perfection. So therefore, that's probably what I look like in heaven. We don't realize that these constructions of beauty are exactly that: they're there to sell you things. And they're created by powerful people who have lots and lots of money to shape how you think. But the Bible doesn't do that. It doesn't give you that kind of information. In fact, it's quite mysterious when it comes to these things. But the apostle Paul in 1 Corinthians 15, when he is talking about the resurrection body, doesn't say that the body will be replaced. He says it'll be transformed.

N. T. Wright points out that something similar goes on in Revelation when the new Jerusalem comes down upon the old Jerusalem. The old Jerusalem is not replaced, it's transformed. There's something about our bodies that we have just now that have some kind of durability, some kind of eternal significance. And the fact that we don't know what that significance entails means that we need to respect everybody irrespective of what you look like, irrespective of the way your body or mind functions. Something about you as a person has durability. When you think about the resurrection in that way, then it has significant implications for how you look at people now. Likewise, the scars Jesus has. If you have a vision of beauty that is perfect in the way that perhaps a magazine will tell you is perfect, then either Jesus' body was imperfect, or we've got something wrong. And I think I'd rather go for the latter.

How do you imagine health? What does health feel and look like to you?

I've been thinking about this word called *homefulness* recently. I found it in a very brief comment by Walter Brueggemann. It's to do with how you feel at home in any given situation. I suppose it's probably linked in with the doctrine of creation – that God created the world and said this is your home. But to have a sense of homefulness means that you have a sense of who you are and why you're here, and that you have some kind of awareness and control over your circumstances. Because home is a place where you find your identity. Home is where you do everything with your family or community. It's a central point.

Homefulness is a concept that, I think, resonates deeply with both health and the vocation of health care workers. To be a healing presence – in the fullest sense – is to become someone with whom others can feel at home. Illness, in so many of its forms, is a kind of exile. It dislocates. It estranges you from your body, from your story, from your community – sometimes even from God. And so, the work of healing must involve more than diagnosis and intervention; it must participate in the work of rehoming. To offer homefulness is to offer presence that is spacious, hospitable, and trustworthy – a space where people feel recognized, safe, and named. It's in that space, even amid ongoing suffering or unresolved symptoms, that people might begin to feel they are coming home – to themselves, to others, and perhaps, in some deep way, to God.

Summer 2025

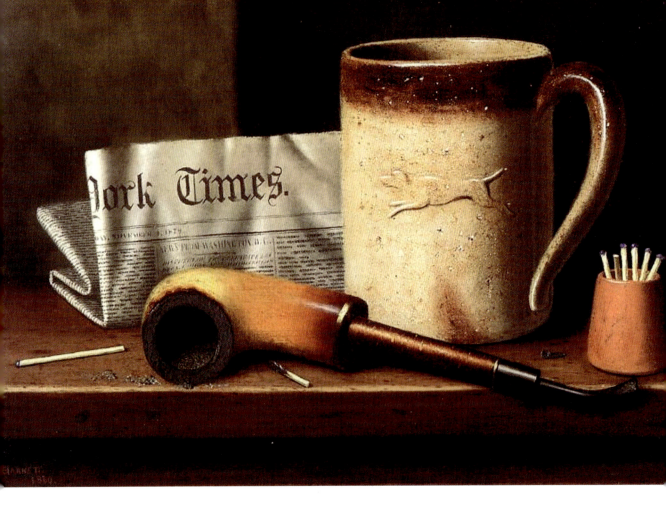

In Defense of Pipe and Pint

*Smoking and drinking carry known risks.
Here's why I haven't given them up.*

MALCOLM GUITE

William Michael Harnett, *His Mug and His Pipe*, oil, 1880.

WE LIVE IN AN AGE when, at least in the affluent West, there is something of an obsession with bodily health, with healthy lifestyles, healthy eating and drinking, and a constant cycle of new diets, regimens, vitamin supplements, and exercise fads. And of course, attendant on these, and fueling their consumer ratings, a rash of hypochondria, self-diagnosis, health scares based on spurious medical blogs, etc. The one thing all these trends, however helpful or harmful, have in common is an essentially mechanistic and reductive account of health or (in the current jargon) "wellness" itself.

It is assumed that the body is essentially a machine, a linked series of mechanical processes whose performance can be optimized by ensuring the best input, in terms of foods and supplements, and the best output in terms of exercise. There is analytic attention to food and drink in terms of nutrients, fiber, and alcohol content, but no consideration of the ambience, culture, atmosphere, nuance, gregarious and social aspects of eating and drinking, no consideration of their meaning or the part they play in the richness, depth, and happiness of human life considered as a whole integrated experience. Most of the advice we are given on how to live a healthy life ignores or even undermines the great intangibles, the unmeasurable *qualities*, as opposed to the measured *quantities*, which make that life worth living.

On the mere input/output analysis, I should give up the convivial evenings in many-storied, oak-raftered pubs, where my friends and I, and often strangers who are welcomed into the circle of conversation, sit for a while and set the world to rights. I should give up the pipes I have collected and smoked over the years, each with its own beautiful pattern of grain, each with its own cluster of stories and memories of solitary musing or wonderful conversation. My body might be technically healthier for the loss, but I contend my whole being, my personhood, my sense of community, of participating in something immemorial, hallowed by the poets, endorsed by the sages, celebrated by almost all my favorite writers, my life, taken as a whole, would be poorer. And if I gave these things up as part of an obsession with my own health, then my attention would have been diverted from others to self, from community to individual, from soul to body, and I would be enclosed in a solipsistic cubicle, constantly taking my own pulse.

In saying this I do not mean to glide hastily over very real concerns about excessive smoking and drinking. There is consensus: smoking poses serious health risks. And many a family has been harmed or destroyed by the disease of alcoholism.

If I thought my pipe or my pint posed a risk to my family's happiness or wholeness, I would give it up in a moment. But I have chosen not to give up pipe and pint. And I have done so because of the sense that I would lose something of a broader health if I did. What would I lose in giving up the pint, the pipe, and the pub? I know no better way of answering this question than in my native tongue: poetry, both my own and that of others. So let me try.

Pub and Pint

In his *Songs of Innocence and of Experience* William Blake often gives voice to the poor and marginalized, the unnoticed and voiceless. In one such poem he speaks from the voice of someone who finds himself more welcome in the pub than the church:

> Dear Mother, dear Mother, the Church is cold,
> But the Ale-house is healthy & pleasant & warm;
> Besides I can tell where I am used well . . .

He goes on later in the poem to say that if church were only as welcoming and nonjudgmental as the alehouse, then:

> modest dame Lurch, who is always at Church,
> Would not have bandy children nor fasting nor birch.

Surprising though it may be to some of my stricter Christian brothers and sisters, there is something of a history of thinking of the church in this way. When Christ tells the parable of the Good Samaritan (Luke 10:25–37), he cannot think of a better place to take the wounded man for healing, until he comes again, than an inn. The early church commentators say the inn in the parable is meant to be a type of the church.

What is it about an inn, what we in England would call "our local," that is so beneficent? It is

---

Malcolm Guite is a poet, singer-songwriter, and author of eight books, including What Do Christians Believe? *and* Sounding the Seasons. *He serves as the chaplain of Girton College at the University of Cambridge, and moonlights as lead singer and guitarist for the blues-rock band Mystery Train.*

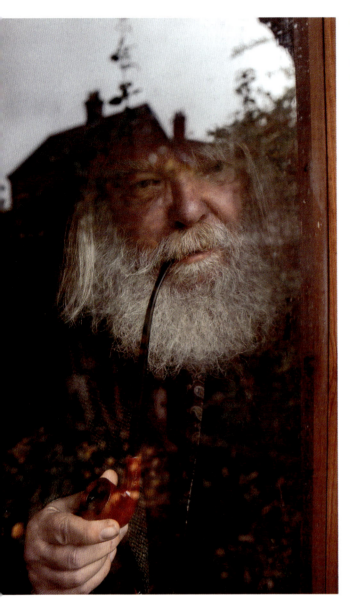

building, it speaks of a continuity across the generations, a solidarity we have with our own past. I reflected on what the public house means to me personally in the unpublished ballade I wrote called "I'll Have Another Pint of Porter Please":

> I love the mullioned snug, the brewers dray
> And all the tapster's tacit craft and lore.
> To reach a village inn when skies are grey,
> To step out of the rain and through the door,
> To feel the warmth, to tread the stone-flagged floor,
> And sit beside the fire and take our ease,
> This is the bliss our little life is for,
> I'll have another pint of porter please.

Ballades (the form popularized by French medieval poet François Villon) traditionally end with an envoy addressed to the prince who is the poet's patron. So, as a Christian, I ended this poem with an envoy to Christ:

> Prince there's an inn that you have kept in store,
> And given to St. Peter both its keys,
> I'm on my way, but tell him, well before,
> I'll have another pint of porter please.

Amid the pub's conviviality, I remember my mortality and I look forward to the resurrection and the banquet of heaven. Now it could be argued, of course, that I could go to the inn and drink fizzy lemonade, but my counterargument would be both that such beverages might be worse for me in the long run than my modest pint, and also that the alcohol in the beer plays its part too, in relaxation, in a sense of ease, in loosening a little the rigid inhibitions which, at least in English culture, keep folk from talking to one another. Of course good drink can be abused with tragic results, but if teetotalism were enforced and all the pubs closed, individual bodies might be healthier in one respect but the unrelieved stress and the epidemic of isolation and loneliness that might ensue, as we found in lockdown when the

open, it is welcoming, it is in every sense a *public house*, which is where the term "pub" comes from. It is therefore a place where different people from the same community, with all their differences of background and politics and personality, can find a convivial space to meet one another. If it happens to be an old inn, then, like the old church

Malcolm Guite, photograph by Betty Laura Zapata.

pubs really did close down, might be far worse for our health than the pints in good company would have been.

Pipe

I turn now to my other forbidden, or at least widely frowned-on, pleasure: the pleasure of smoking my pipe. I concede that I am on shakier ground here. I don't dispute the clear and consistent evidence that smoking is harmful in the long run and that it is linked to cancer. However, I would note that pipe smoking is distinct from cigarette smoking in that the pipe smoker does not inhale the smoke but merely tastes and savors it, then breathes it out again. There is then a risk for me, if a comparatively small one. Why do I take that risk? Again, it is because I set the physical aspect of my health in the context of my whole health and welfare, in the context of what it means to flourish.

Like my pint, my pipe carries with it a whole penumbra of literary and personal associations, and smoking it always means that I am relaxing my tensions, letting go of my stresses, savoring life and the present moment in all its fullness. Given my high blood pressure and the general stresses of life, even my doctor might concede that this genial relaxation, this easing and letting go of tensions, is just the thing I need. Again, I can best express the experience of my risky behavior in the form of poetry, also in the ballade form:

Smoke Rings from My Pipe

All the long day's weariness is done
I'm free at last to do just as I will,
Take out my pipe, admire the setting sun,
Practice the art of simply sitting still.
Thank God I have this briar bowl to fill,
I leave the world with all its hopeless hype,
Its pressures, and its ever-ringing till,
And let it go in smoke rings from my pipe.

The hustle and the bustle, these I shun,
The tasks that trouble and the cares that kill,
The false idea that there's a race to run,
The pushing of that weary stone uphill,
The wretched iPhone's all-insistent trill,
Whingers and whiners, each with their own gripe,
I pack them in tobacco leaves until
They're blown away in smoke rings from my pipe.

And then at last my real work is begun:
My chance to chant, to exercise the skill
Of summoning the muses, one by one,
To meet me in their temple, touch my quill,
(I have a pen but quills are better still)
And when the soul is full, the time is ripe,
Kindle the fire of poetry that will
Breathe and expand like smoke rings from my pipe.

The Psalm says "Man is like a breath" (144:4), and as I watch the smoke from my pipe evaporate in the air, I am reminded of this reality. And perhaps this is the founding answer as to why I still smoke my pipe. Try as we may to optimize our bodies like machines, we cannot escape death except through resurrection. A good life is not merely one indefinitely extended through meticulous attention to bodily wellness, but one spent in community and with joy. For some this may mean giving up pipe and pint, if they pose a distraction or a risk to that conviviality with family and friends, or to their own holistically considered health. But for me, risks though there may be, pipes and pints have helped bring me back into that convivial circle of life, and given me moments of connection, of rest, of wonder in a world often fraught and disconnected. This is a choice I make, aware of risks, but without fear. And so I end again with an envoy addressed to Christ.

Prince, I have done with grinding at the mill,
These petty-pelting tyrants aren't my type,
So lift me up and set me on a hill,
A free man blowing smoke rings from his pipe.

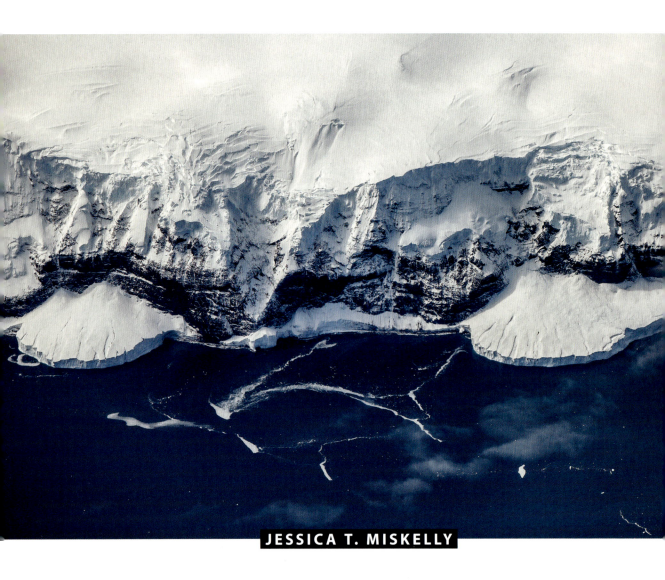

JESSICA T. MISKELLY

Of Antarctic Ice *and* Ocean Currents

On an icebreaker in the Weddell Sea, I felt a warming planet's pulse.

THE SUN SKIMS LOW on the horizon as I snatch wakefully for the midnight alarm. Sleep is hard when it's never dark. Unthreading safety straps, I roll out off the top bunk to the roiling floor, scratchy commercial carpet pitching on the wilds of the Southern Ocean. The stabilizer screeches like a demonic playground swing as it throws the ship back the opposite direction from the lurch of a wave. Foam laces the porthole, glinting over ink-slush seas.

Aerial photo of Antarctica's coastline by Matt Palmer, 2017.

That's a memory from 2007, when I sailed on Australia's now-retired icebreaker, the *Aurora Australis*, as part of a scientific research voyage monitoring oceans and biology around Antarctica. My role involved collecting water samples to monitor changes (potentially due to climate change) in water properties around the continent.

During the last deglaciation fifteen thousand years ago, global sea level rose nearly sixty feet in less than five hundred years. Known as meltwater pulse 1A, this event was discovered in 1989 via shallow-dwelling corals found in the deep sea, bolstering emerging theories that climate change could be rapid. Ice and sediment cores in Greenland had already revealed evidence of recurrent spikes in atmospheric temperature of 10 to 15 degrees Celsius during the last sixty thousand years, and these spikes were closely spaced in time with other sea-level rise events. Ice sheet formation and decay clearly played a role in these climate changes, and the game was on to determine how, and how much. As a newly minted scientist, I wanted to play.

The ice sheets over North America and Europe disappeared around ten thousand years ago, leaving just Greenland behind. Antarctica has been steadier. Cut off from the rest of the world thirty-four million years ago when the passage between the tip of South America and the Antarctic Peninsula opened at the same time global atmospheric CO_2 levels were decreasing, Antarctica has become a runaway train of ice accumulation. The circumpolar ocean acts like a flywheel, flinging out much of the heat from further north that tries to penetrate south. While fossils from the Eocene period fifty million years ago reveal lush vegetation in Antarctica, ice sheets one to three miles thick now cover much of the continent, locking up water that would otherwise be in the ocean. Antarctica is the largest ice mass on the planet, containing enough water to raise global sea level by more than 160 feet. For comparison, Greenland has an ice mass equivalent to around a twenty-three-foot global sea-level rise.

Yet sea-level rise projections from the Intergovernmental Panel on Climate Change did not, until recently, include the effects of melting ice sheets. This is because the dynamics of ice sheet accumulation and decay are nonlinear and hard to quantify. So, while we understand many individual effects – for example, we know that ice melts when it is warmer, that warmth is driven by increases in greenhouse gases, and that heat takes time to reach Antarctica – we don't fully understand how these different effects, or drivers, interact, at least not in exact, quantifiable ways. The effect of a small push from one driver can be largely unnoticeable. But if all the pushes line up in the same direction or pass a certain threshold, they can start to reinforce each other and become runaway. Prediction certainty from complex nonlinear systems is low.

Scientists like me are drawn to such intricate systems and, despite common perceptions from nonscientists, seeking to understand our world need not be a domineering or disenchanting pursuit. The act of witnessing, examining, and attempting to comprehend the vast complexity of the natural world often leads scientists to experiences of awe and wonder, congruent with religious experiences or what others feel in the presence of great art. Awe inspires. Its experience, writes Alister McGrath in *The Territories of Human Reason*, "creates a new receptivity towards increasing understanding, thus offering a powerful stimulus to the scientific engagement with nature." This engagement need not demand complete and total knowledge. For Einstein, nature's "magnificent structure" was something

---

Jessica T. Miskelly lives in the Southern Highlands of Australia. She has a master's degree in climate science from the University of New South Wales and has worked as a meteorologist since 2003.

"we can only grasp imperfectly," and most scientists would agree. We're not all cold, calculating types. But we try to understand.

Orbital Cycles

Of course, continuing a decade of shiftwork, I got assigned to nightshift on the icebreaking research vessel. Except it wasn't dark. The tilt of the Earth aims the poles toward the sun, so it's always daytime there in summer. A particularly warm summer can result in more ice melt than normal. Less ice decreases reflectivity, allowing the region to absorb more heat, which melts more ice. Maybe, argues a leading theory, so much melt would occur that the next winter could not re-accumulate all the lost ice. The whole ice sheet could melt over a series of warm seasons. Alternatively, successive colder seasons could lead to snow cover persisting through summer to eventually become permanent ice sheets.

We know that summers and winters are periodically warmer or colder due to cyclical changes in the Earth's orbit known as Milankovitch cycles. Eccentricity, where the Earth's orbit alternately squashes and unsquashes like a wire ring, and obliquity, where the tilt of the Earth waxes and wanes, are dominant, enhancing or weakening seasons. Long-term geological records of ice and temperature trends clearly follow these cycles. Less clear is why climate history reflects these cycles more strongly or weakly at different times and why one is sometimes more dominant than another.

Carbon Cycles

Cycles surround us. Overlaid on the push of orbital cycles are the pushes of atmospheric greenhouse gas concentrations. CO_2, a major greenhouse gas, cycles through animals, plants, the Earth's crust, and oceans over the millennia, becoming trapped as tiny air bubbles in ice and leaving markers in sediment from which climate scientists can take core samples. CO_2 blankets the Earth to varying degrees, preventing the day-to-night temperature swings of over 100 degrees Celsius that happen on Mars.

Oceans, in particular, absorb great masses of CO_2 and transport it downward in deep vertical currents to the "carbon sink," preventing, at least initially, atmospheric CO_2 from rising as high as it would otherwise. Here, CO_2 is deposited and buried on the ocean bed. Or CO_2 may outgas from the ocean when the water returns to the surface hundreds to thousands of years later.

The marine surveyors send down a camera. We watch crinoids in real-time bounce like orange long-haired wigs, breathing in oxygen that the ocean currents have taken down.

The Earth breathes.

Ocean Cycles

And the icy poles are the lungs. Ocean ventilation cycles are directly driven by the icy polar regions since that is where water gets coldest. Cold water is denser than warm water. Salt water is denser than freshwater. Cold, salty water is densest. If sufficiently dense, it sinks – kind of like the opposite of "warm air rises." It is convection in reverse but in the oceans not the air. Salinity is key, as it affects water density more strongly than temperature. Without sufficient salinity, water can't cool below the temperature required to give it the density to sink, and our oceans stagnate.

In Antarctica, the source of salinity is freezing sea-ice. Since freshwater preferentially freezes over saltwater at the same temperature, the formation of abundant sea-ice like that which we were breaking through each day (always I thought of Shackleton's ship, stuck fast till the ice squeezed it to crumpling point) leaves behind water that is saltier than the original. Then, this salty water left behind by forming sea-ice sinks. Deep under the Weddell and Ross Seas, it waterfalls off the continental shelf to the abyssal plain four miles below and spreads north, one part of the global ocean ventilation. Antarctic Bottom Water (AABW) is the deepest deepwater in the world and it's why we

Photograph courtesy of Jessica Miskelly.

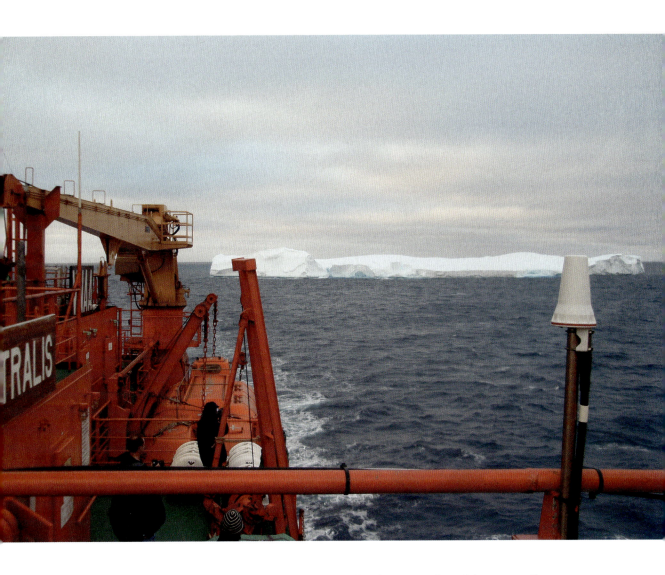

were here: we wanted to see if its composition and formation rate were indicative of healthy breath.

Flickering screens line the CTD (Conductivity, Temperature, Depth) control room and a computer bank sits in the middle. At 1:00 a.m. the CTD night shift leader, Mark, professionally explains the intricacies of sample collection. Thus prepared, we don oilskin overalls and boots and thwump to the wet room to prepare the CTD rosette, which looks like a bunch of gas cylinders arranged on a circular rig. A giant winch hook punctures the top middle. Once prepared, the rig is secured to a chain and the ship's crew takes over, craning it out from the ship's side, then lowering it through heaving swell.

Back in the control room, a walkie-talkie code of "slow," "hold," "stop" guides the rosette down to gently bump bottom. Then it's pulled up in stages, stopping at predetermined levels to tap a key and pop off a cylinder top that lets water in. When it's back on board, we quickly extract samples of water. Erlenmeyer flasks full and hands numb – hurry, the onboard hydrochemist wants to analyze the samples immediately – pinpoints of data to which we try to fit nets of understanding.

There's a lot of data collection and categorizing before glamorous theorizing.

The author's observational ship in Antarctica, 2007.

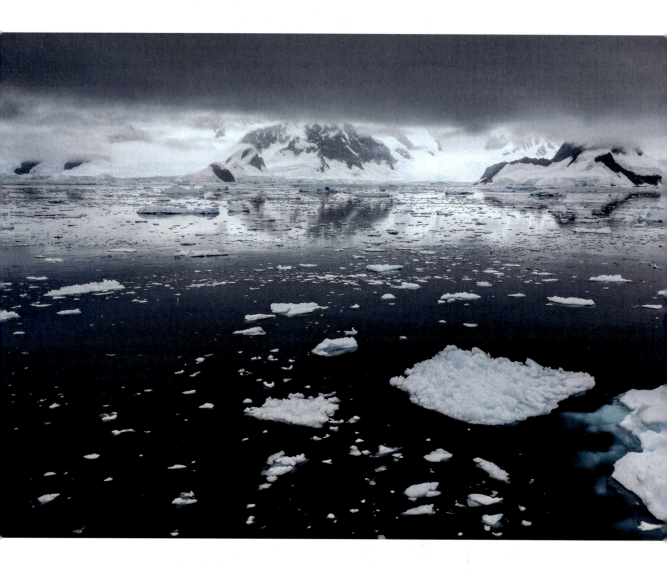

Ventilating deepwater also forms in the Northern Hemisphere, specifically in the North Atlantic, where it is known as North Atlantic Deepwater (NADW). Here, the essential salinity is supplied via the Gulf Stream and North Atlantic currents from near-tropical areas further south. These ventilating currents in the Northern and Southern Hemispheres connect in the depths: a great conveyer of water, salt, dissolved gases, suspended particles, and heat. Together, AABW and NADW complete a circuit of ocean ventilation – the ocean breathes.

And it can stop.

Oceans as Climate Modulator or Amplifier

In the late 1980s, scientists examining sediment cores from the ocean floor noticed patterns that indicated NADW had been much weaker in the past. Now, it is widely accepted that there was at least one NADW shutdown during the last glacial period. This backed up a theoretical model that an oceanographer named Henry Stommel had advanced in the early 1960s.

Stommel hypothesized that when the source of salinity is remote (way back in the equatorial Atlantic), it is possible to create a feedback loop:

Wilhelmina Bay on the Antarctic Peninsula, 2017.

freshen North Atlantic surface water (by melting a nearby ice sheet, say) and it becomes less dense, so deepwater sinking slows. Once sinking slows, less warm, salty surface water is drawn northward, which leads to further freshening in the North Atlantic. Sinking then slows further, and the slowdown becomes self-feeding. With sufficient freshwater, the overall circulation system (known as Atlantic Meridional Overturning Circulation, or AMOC) can come to a near standstill.

The North Atlantic currents are what moderate the climate of lands around the North Atlantic. Western Europe, in particular, and the northeastern United States have a much milder climate than Siberia or inland Canada thanks to the Gulf Stream and North Atlantic currents. A stalled AMOC disrupts global heat distribution. Temperatures over Greenland could drop as much as 10 degrees Celsius, with lesser drops of an estimated 2 to 5 degrees in western Europe and near the northeastern United States, strongly dependent on the accompanying atmospheric CO_2 concentration. Areas to the south would become much warmer, the contrast likely driving unprecedented weather events. Note that these are annual average temperatures; extremes, which are more noticeable and have a greater effect on life, would change even more. Many climate scientists believe there is a non-negligible risk of an AMOC shutdown happening over the coming century.

Why Bother Monitoring?

The AMOC is considered so vital that it has been continuously monitored since 2004. Hundreds of sensors are strung like lights across the ocean to record temperature, salinity, and other parameters indicative of strength. There are signs of a decrease.

It's fair to question the point of such monitoring. I often wonder myself. What do we do if we see signs of an imminent collapse?

In meteorology, observations allow us to forecast extreme weather events so people can take action. But in longer-term climate modeling, it's unlikely we'll do anything in response to a dire forecast, at least given our track record in combating climate change so far. Are we demanding to know everything before we do anything? Are we forgetting to be awestruck by what we already know?

Antarctic Bottom Water is also monitored, though not continuously. Back in 2007, I was researching how stable AABW was, to anticipate how much it might be affected by possible human-induced climate changes. It's less susceptible than

It's fair to question the point of this monitoring. I often wonder myself. What do we do if we see signs of an imminent collapse?

NADW. Persistent winds tend to push surface freshwater away north, sea-ice removes surface freshwater as it freezes, and sufficiently salty water still manages to sink. It is not completely invulnerable, though. Observations from repeat samplings over recent decades show warming, freshening, and reduced formation rates. The combined effects of atmospheric warming and warm water encroaching south are destabilizing ice sheets.

The ice sheet in West Antarctica – the part with the elbow-like peninsula – is most vulnerable to collapse because a lot of it is not grounded; it fans out between underlying rocky peninsulas, linking across large tracts of ocean. The East Antarctic Ice Sheet is more stable but also reaches out into the ocean in vast ice shelves, where it is vulnerable to basal melting from warming oceans. In 2002, the Larsen B ice shelf – the size of Long Island – shocked scientists by collapsing into the ocean over just a few weeks. In 2022, the Conger ice shelf – a bit smaller than Rome – collapsed. The Greenland ice sheet is also showing clear signs of weakening.

The Earth's climate changed drastically in the prehuman past as well. Cycles have been plowing on for millennia. But it's also clearly a finely balanced system. So, while it's true there is high uncertainty around the exact response of ice sheets and ocean currents to changing climate, there is high certainty that they *do* respond.

The demand for more certainty around the exact impacts of climate change before taking action is a common refrain. I'm less sympathetic than I was; certainty is a mirage, and it's worth remembering we don't have perfect predictive power or understanding in other fields either. Sometimes, the public seems more demanding of certainty than the scientists.

Will We Change?

I am tired of being asked to justify my "opinion" on climate change. None of us is completely impartial, but evidence is not opinion. Even in meteorology, where I have worked for the last fifteen years, I can't avoid climate questions and find myself making more frequent "unprecedented" forecasts compared to past years.

So, knowing what I do, do I live as I know one should? I'm too small to make a difference to climate change, after all, probably, right?

But what we do at home seeps into the world at large, whether it's our energy usage and carbon footprint, or acts and attitudes of hypocrisy and nihilism.

We don't get to jettison personal responsibility just because governments and corporations let us down.

In Australia, we live in houses bigger than ever before, which require more energy to heat and cool and rarely consider passive solar design, which allows warming sun inside in winter but blocks it in summer. Air-conditioning use has skyrocketed – so much for the Australian reputation of being good with the heat. In the Northern Hemisphere, meanwhile, in winter we are heating homes so far above ambient that we barely need long sleeves. The International Energy Agency found that turning the thermostat down just one degree could cut European gas demand by 7 percent.

Living in a way that is sustainable, rather than stripping our world to within an inch of what we can get away with, is an act of creation care. It is also an act of loving our neighbor: those living on low-lying islands or in overcrowded cities who can't afford air conditioning, heating, or flood insurance will be the most immediately affected by climate change. It is also the appropriate response to awareness of our smallness in the face of vastness, an acceptance of the fact that the world is not ours to consume, control, or even fully comprehend. For scientists, this calls for scientific humility that counters Enlightenment promises of one day understanding everything and hence, in a sense, bringing the world to heel. For Christians, it is one more call to hold together the knowledge that we are never fully in control with the command to act nevertheless. We should not despise "the day of small things" (Zech. 4:10) in which we live, nor languish in inaction waiting for God to do big things.

In January this year, European scientists extracted the longest continuous ice core to date, the bottom portion containing trapped air bubbles and particles that are over one million years old and possibly up to two million years old. Analysis will reveal some climate secrets and leave us in awe of the complexity of our world, but others will remain secret. The scientists and the rest of us will go home, and we will all have to keep living as best we can as the planet moves, the CO_2 cycles turn, the oceans breathe, and the ice creaks and heaves in response.

READINGS

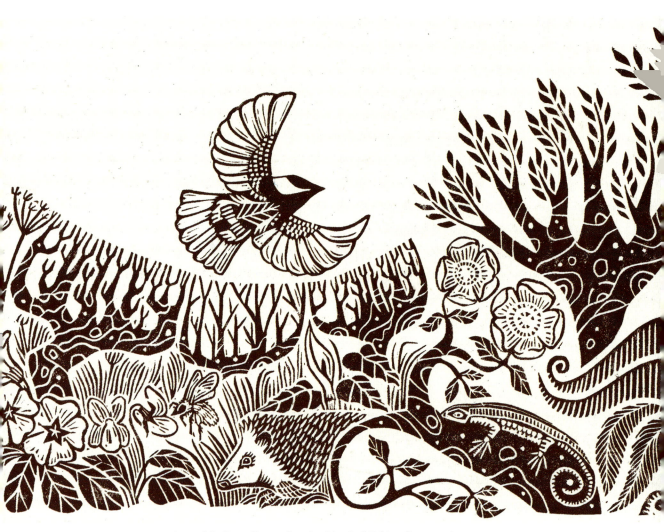

Artwork by Becca Thorne, from her *Marginal Habitats* linocut series.

Health Is Belonging

Four thinkers stretch our understanding of disease and its remedy.

Edith Stein ♦ *Wendell Berry*
Teresa of Ávila ♦ *Christoph Friedrich Blumhardt*

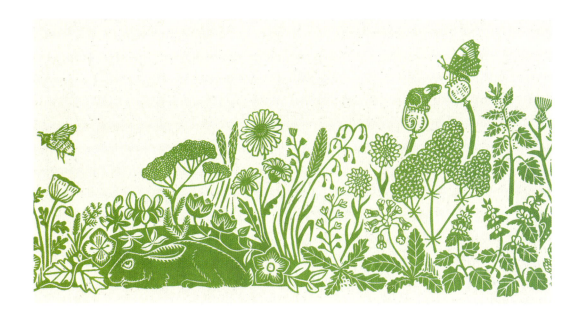

Edith Stein (1891–1942) came from an Orthodox Jewish family. At the age of thirty she converted to Catholicism, and she later took vows as a Carmelite nun. Because of her Jewish ancestry she was executed at Auschwitz by the Nazis in August 1942.

THE SOUL IS HOUSED in a body on whose vigor and health its own vigor and health depend – even if not exclusively nor simply. On the other hand, the body receives its nature as body – life, motion, form, gestalt, and spiritual significance – through the soul. The world of the spirit is founded on sensuousness, which is spiritual as much as physical: the intellect, knowing its activity to be rational, reveals a world; the will intervenes creatively and formatively in this world; the emotion receives this world inwardly and puts it to the test. But the extent and relationship of these powers vary from one individual to another, and particularly from man to woman. . . .

But a certain danger is involved here. If the correct, natural order is to exist between soul and body (i.e., the order as it corresponds to unfallen nature), then the necessary nourishment, care, and exercise must be provided for the healthy organism's smooth function. As soon as more physical satisfaction is given to the body, and it corresponds to its corrupted nature to demand more, then it results in a decline of spiritual existence. Instead of controlling and spiritualizing the body, the soul is controlled by it; and the body loses accordingly in its character as a human body. The more intimate the relationship of the soul and body is, just so will the danger of the spiritual decline be greater.

Edith Stein, *Essays on Woman* v. 2 revised second edition (ICS Publications: Institute of Carmelite Studies, 1996). Used by permission.

About the artist: Becca Thorne is a British illustrator and linocut printmaker. Her work focuses on themes of wildlife, nature, history, and folklore, with a particular emphasis on conservation. Her *Marginal Habitats* series, shown here, explores the diversity of interconnected flora and fauna that make up healthy ecosystems.

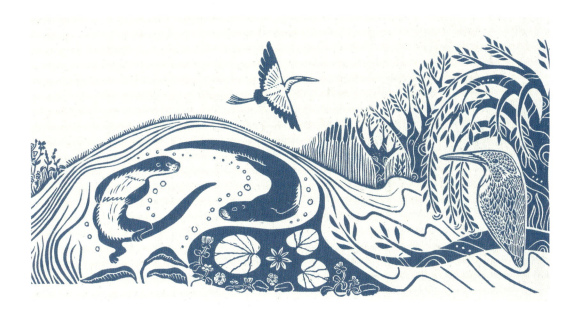

Wendell Berry (b. 1934) is an American novelist, poet, essayist, environmental activist, cultural critic, and farmer.

IN HEALING, THE BODY is restored to itself. It begins to live again by its own powers and instincts, to the extent that it can do so. To the extent that it can do so, it goes free of drugs and mechanical helps. Its appetites return. It relishes food and rest. The patient is restored to family and friends, home and community and work.

This process has a certain naturalness and inevitability, like that by which a child grows up, but industrial medicine seems to grasp it only tentatively and awkwardly. For example, any ordinary person would assume that a place of healing would put a premium upon rest, but hospitals are notoriously difficult to sleep in. They are noisy all night, and the routine interventions go on relentlessly. The body is treated as a machine that does not need to rest. . . .

In the world of love, things separated by efficiency and specialization strive to come back together. And yet love must confront death, and accept it, and learn from it. Only in confronting death can earthly love learn its true extent, its immortality. Any definition of health that is not silly must include death. The world of love includes death, suffers it, and triumphs over it. The world of efficiency is defeated by death; at death, all its instruments and procedures stop. The world of love continues, and of this grief is the proof.

Wendell Berry, excerpt from "Health is Membership" from *The Art of the Commonplace: The Agrarian Essays*. Copyright © 1994, 2002 by Wendell Berry. Reprinted with the permission of The Permissions Company, LLC on behalf of Counterpoint Press.

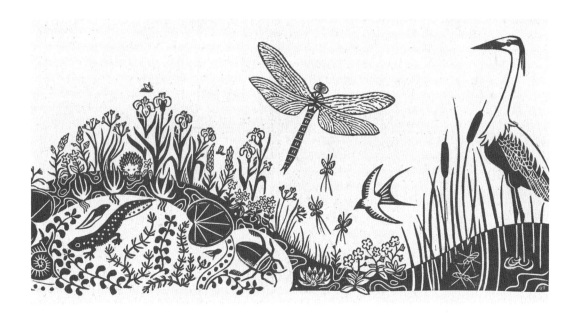

Teresa of Ávila (1515–1582) was a Spanish nun and mystic. The originator of the Carmelite Reform, she was the first woman to be honored as a doctor of the church.

ALL THESE TOKENS of the fear of God came to me through prayer; and the greatest of them was this, that fear was swallowed up of love – for I never thought of chastisement. All the time I was so ill, my strict watch over my conscience reached to all that is mortal sin.

O my God! I wished for health, that I might serve Thee better; that was the cause of all my ruin. For when I saw how helpless I was through paralysis, being still so young, and how the physicians of this world had dealt with me, I determined to ask those of heaven to heal me – for I wished, nevertheless, to be well, though I bore my illness with great joy. Sometimes, too, I used to think that if I recovered my health, and yet were lost forever, I was better as I was. But, for all that, I thought I might serve God much better if I were well. This is our delusion; we do not resign ourselves absolutely to the disposition of our Lord, who knows best what is for our good. . . .

I know not how we can wish to live, seeing that everything is so uncertain. Once, O Lord, I thought it impossible to forsake thee so utterly; and now that I have forsaken thee so often, I cannot help being afraid; for when thou didst withdraw but a little from me, I fell down to the ground at once. Blessed forever be thou! Though I have forsaken thee, thou hast not forsaken me so utterly but that thou hast come again and raised me up, giving me thy hand always.

Teresa of Ávila, *The Life of St. Teresa of Jesus* (London: Thomas Baker, 1904).

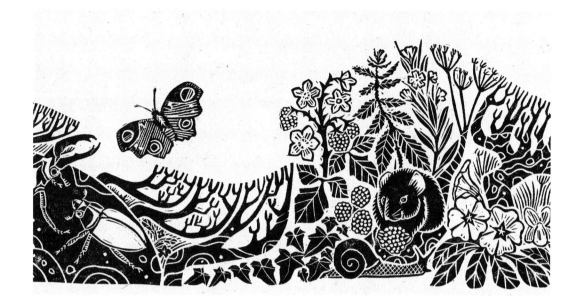

Christoph Friedrich Blumhardt (1842–1919) was a pastor in Bad Boll, Germany.

There are two sides to the gospel of Jesus Christ. It is a message of forgiveness of sins, of everlasting life, but also a message of opposition to human misery. Not only is an end to sin proclaimed, but also an end to suffering and death. All suffering shall cease! Just as sin is overcome through the blood of Christ, so suffering will come to an end at the resurrection. When Jesus performed signs and wonders, he was proclaiming the gospel against suffering.

With this gospel we can be certain that the wretchedness of this world will cease, just as we are sure of everlasting life. We cannot separate these two sides of Christ. We must not one-sidedly emphasize the cross and forgiveness, while ignoring the resurrection and the overcoming of our misery. It is Satan's trick to try and make us waver so that the Savior does not receive a full and complete hearing.

Faced with the world's longing for redemption, it is obvious that we can never bring real comfort through the gospel as long as we stress only the one thing – that the Savior forgives our sins – and otherwise the world can go its own way. Similarly, we would be unable to bring real comfort through the gospel, if we represented the Savior only as a miracle-worker and proclaimed, "Be comforted, you can be healed through the Savior." Then repentance and forgiveness would be utterly forgotten, and no fundamental change would ever take place in people.

Jesus allowed the sick to come to him, just as he did sinners. He was ready to forgive sins and ready to heal. There were times when very few sinners came, only sick people. And Jesus welcomed them all. Oh, that the nations would hear the good news! That the sick would come, and that sinners would come – all are welcome!"

Christoph Friedrich Blumhardt, *The God Who Heals* (Plough Publishing House, 2016).

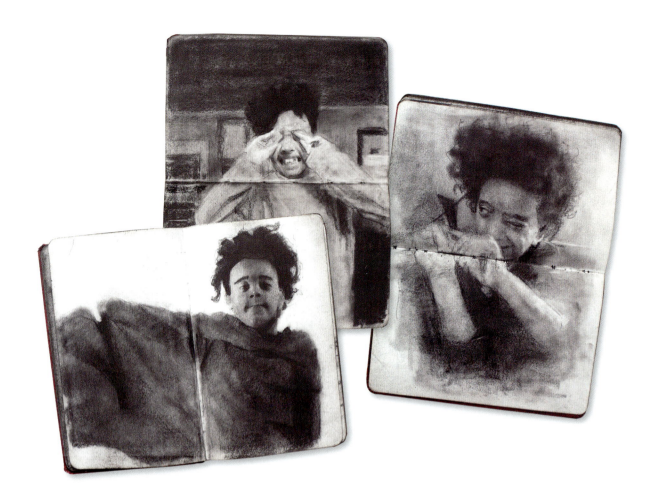

What Families with Autistic Children Know

For parents of neurodiverse children, church and school can be another hurdle.

SAM TOMLIN

ON A ROAD TRIP a few summers ago, our family drove through North Wales to enjoy a few days with our three children. Such outings aren't unusual for us; our homeschooling curriculum gives us freedom to occasionally take a few days off for fun as well as education. Returning home to Liverpool, we stopped at a playground to run around a little before climbing back in the car. It was a school day, so the park was deserted except for a mother and her son. This mother was trying to have a phone conversation while her son tugged incessantly at her sleeve. This went on for five minutes or so, as they drifted toward us. Seeing that the

All artwork by Jerry Montoya.

mother was in distress, we invited the child to play a game with our children. When she finished her call, they came over.

Almost as soon as he approached, we could tell that this child was autistic. I do not say that lightly, but as parents of an autistic child ourselves, we have come to recognize the probable signs. In a striking way, this boy was like our son, exhibiting many identical mannerisms: the way he moved his hands when he was speaking, the intonations of his voice, the lack of eye contact, and, tellingly, the constant clawing at his exasperated mother. In his mother's eyes we recognized a look mirrored by many parents of neurodiverse children: a combination of utter despair and stoic determination. Being a parent of any child is hard at times, but when your child does not fit into the prescribed societal standards of "normality," it is almost impossible to communicate the pain to someone who hasn't been there.

As we shared conversation, this mother told us she had taken her son out of mainstream education due to bullying. Every morning had involved a meltdown and a point-blank refusal to go. She had to leave her job, which led to increased financial pressures, and with no teaching experience or family nearby, she felt completely out of her depth trying to educate her son. On top of this, her husband had taken to alcohol partly due to the challenges of raising their son. Almost every day, she would trail around the parks, counting down the hours until bedtime offered a momentary respite. We spoke for almost half an hour; she and my wife exchanged numbers, but we never heard from her again.

Hers is not an uncommon story. As members of various social media groups for parents of neurodiverse children, we see numerous posts a day from parents (mostly mothers) who are on the point of despair. They write of children refusing school, making life difficult for siblings, rendering simple trips and social occasions almost impossible to navigate, and putting pressure on marriages. In our experience this "community" is one often marked by exhaustion, loneliness, discouragement at relatives who misunderstand or downplay the condition, deep anxiety, and high levels of family breakdown.

About the artist: Jerry Montoya is a Colombian American artist whose work often features his son, who has autism. "Autism in our house means giggles and hugs, frustration and tears. It means strangers giving looks, and even closest friends not quite understanding. . . . It means an intelligent, unique, silly little boy and a house full of love."

I T SHOULD NOT HAVE TO be this way. Western societies are beginning a wider conversation about neurodiversity. While some autistic people challenge its association with disability, autism is described by the UK National Autistic Society as a "lifelong developmental disability which affects how people communicate and interact with the world." Serious research began in the early twentieth century when it was estimated that about one in a couple of thousand people were autistic. Some estimates today suggest approximately one in fifty. It is often said that if you meet one autistic person, you meet one autistic person; that is, that generalizing about autism can be dangerous. The UK National Autistic Society suggests, however, that certain characteristics may be more common in autistic people: social communication and interaction challenges; repetitive and restrictive behavior; and

---

Captain Sam Tomlin is an officer in the Salvation Army. He and his wife, Jenni, lead Stoneycroft Salvation Army Community Church in Liverpool, United Kingdom, where they live with their three children.

over- or under-sensitivity to light, sound, taste, or touch.

It is unsurprising, therefore, that autistic people often find life difficult in a world that does not accommodate their needs. Western society prizes self-possession and self-fulfillment. Whether we like it or not, being liked and "fitting in" go

---

Perhaps we inadvertently picture heaven as a place where everyone will be socially adept and accepted, acceptable.

---

a long way toward producing what is horribly phrased "social capital." People like people with social capital: celebrities exhibit it, advertisements promote it, workplaces and areas of social encounter value it.

If you exhibit many of the characteristics often associated with autism, chances are that society will lend you less social capital. The very term "autism" comes from the Greek *autos* (self) and denotes a sense of being self-contained, unable to relate to others well or pick up normative social cues. While research is developing, statistics back up the assumption that autistic people do find the world more difficult to navigate. In the United Kingdom, autistic children are more than twice as likely to be excluded from school than their peers, and more than half do not have access to a quiet space at school or someone to turn to if they need support. Lack of such options impacts parents and caregivers immeasurably.

I HAVE OFTEN THOUGHT about that woman and her son. What does the good news of the gospel and the kingdom of God mean to them? Writer Steve Silberman asserts, "the notion that the cure for the most disabling aspects of autism will never be found in a pill, but in supportive communities, is one that parents have been coming to on their own for generations." As a Christian parent of an autistic child, I think (or hope) that the church should be able to model this best. At times, I have seen glimpses of this – churches going out of their way to cater to the needs of neurodiverse people, perhaps providing sensory rooms if people need to step away, not making a fuss if a child melts down in the middle of a service, or providing sacrificial pastoral care and respite for families who don't know where to turn.

But church understanding of neurodivergence is often limited, and there is sometimes a lingering sense that "difficult children" should be contained so as not to disrupt things too much. There are too many stories of families being asked to leave churches because of disruptive children, and when autism is brought up, the question of "healing" is often close to the surface.

Grant Macaskill, a scholar who helped found the Centre for Autism and Theology at Aberdeen University, says it should not surprise us if the church is not automatically a haven for autistic people and their families. In his book *Autism and the Church*, he writes, "The church is not a safe place just because it is the church. It is not a place where the values of God's kingdom are straightforwardly implemented and applied to the welfare of each member. It is the place where the battle of the flesh and the Spirit occurs most violently, and it may, therefore, continue to be full of dangers for its vulnerable members."

It might be tempting to leave it there, allowing families to roll the dice and hope to find a church that welcomes rather than shames them. Neurodiversity may seem just one more thing to worry about for beleaguered pastors, something to consider alongside other worthy causes. I am the pastor of a local church, and I understand these pressures. My perspective may be skewed

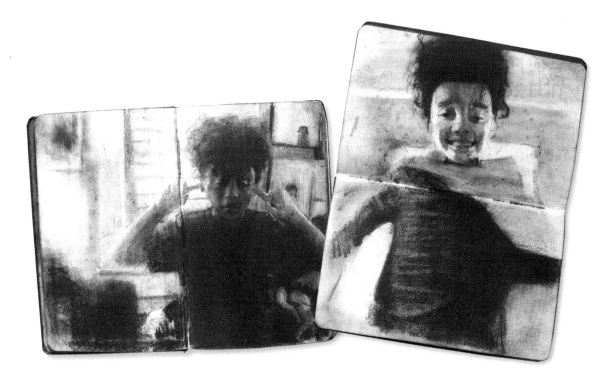

by having an autistic child of my own, but as my understanding has grown, it has opened my eyes to the internal dynamics of a church. I have come to believe that many misunderstandings, squabbles, pressures, and lifelong feelings of shame and rejection are either directly or indirectly associated with neurodiversity.

Macaskill reminds us that this cuts right to the heart of the gospel: "The God of Israel, incarnate in Jesus Christ, is disdainful of the kinds of social or symbolic capital that we consider to be so important, and always has been: he draws near to those we naturally consider to be marginal or even contemptible and elects them to involvement in his work of salvation." Such thoughts have profound implications for the church.

It's natural to be drawn to those who are likable, who demonstrate worth by performing their social function well. Those with autism are, says Macaskill, "not *always* easy to like, they do not always bring much social capital, they may have little utilitarian value to the community." This is not to say that autistic people should be placed on a pedestal of romanticized moral perfection; they can be "genuinely hurtful to those around them and genuinely selfish, in ways that are shaped by their neurotype." In Christian language, they are capable of sin and in need of repentance like everyone else.

In his book *Wondrously Wounded: Theology, Disability, and the Body of Christ,* Macaskill's colleague and leading disability theologian Brian Brock contends that we must "wrench the idea of disability out of its etymological linkage with lack and brokenness." Brock's son Adam, who has autism and Down syndrome, has helped him understand that disability can expose faulty modes of human living; it is acutely linked to our perception of the world and how we relate to each other. The Western view with its narrow understanding of freedom and autonomy easily sneaks into Christian accounts of what it means to be human; perhaps we inadvertently picture heaven as a place where everyone will be socially adept, acceptable, and accepted. This belief implies that neurodiverse conditions are something from which people should be healed.

On a secular level, the belief that autistic people cannot live a full and thriving life lurks behind compassionate arguments for assisted suicide.

Summer 2025

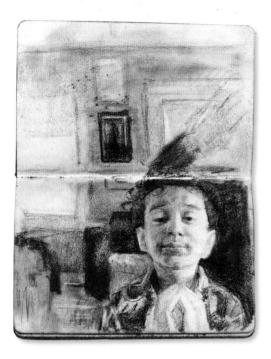

The United Kingdom recently took a significant step toward legalizing assisted dying despite over 350 disability groups warning against such a decision. As I have written previously, evidence from countries such as the Netherlands demonstrates that "suffering" can be seen as an inherent part of being autistic, something that can automatically qualify someone to be euthanized. In some strange way, death is the secular equivalent of Christian understanding of heavenly healing: the deceased may finally "rest in peace."

In his pushback against these assumptions, Brock outlines a more faithful Christian account of flourishing, less to do with bodily healing in the future, and more to do with the new social order that is *already* being established by the Holy Spirit. Reflecting on his life with Adam, Brock names the paradox for many parents of autistic children: the coexistence of frustration and enjoyment, and the gradual realization that your child exposes some of the unhealthy aspects of your own life:

> Adam draws me into his time. His is a much slower time, which does not mean less full of joy or activity, but it is more spatially and conceptually limited and occupied in ways that are constantly cross-grained to expectation. It takes time to learn his ways of behaving, what he enjoys, and how to help him enjoy things.

Our homeschooling schedule often puts me in a park on a weekday afternoon; the gnawing feeling of guilt that I am not being productive has dissipated over time. My son has taught me to live less frantically – I don't have to fill every moment with self-improving action. Relentless productivity, it turns out, is not a fruit of the Spirit. This also helps me as a pastor to reconceive what social relations might look like in the church: not a community that mimics a talk show with socially adept Hollywood A-listers, but truly a fellowship of sinners redeemed by grace, who often hurt or annoy each other, but somehow move toward forgiveness and grace, together.

But there is a danger here, perhaps best expressed by theologian Laura MacGregor. Reflecting on her experience of caring for her son with profound and visible intellectual and physical disabilities, MacGregor recounts how often she was upheld as a paragon of virtue, handpicked by God to prophetically speak deep truths drawn from what she had learned through caregiving. Her reality, however, was very different:

> My day-to-day life was chaotic and overwhelming as I struggled to provide twenty-four-hour care with little respite for Matthew, while also parenting my two typically developing children. My faith crumbled as I cared for an increasingly complex and medically vulnerable child. Despite my community's unfailing ability to locate the Divine in my story, God felt absent. . . . Attempts to honestly discuss my confusion were quickly silenced with theodicies assuring God's goodness and concern.

MacGregor draws on sociologist Arthur Frank, who suggests three types of narrative when it comes to disability: restitution (returning to full health), quest (while no "cure" is found, the protagonist engages in a journey of positive transformation), and chaos (no meaningful resolution, and therefore threatening). Despite people thrusting a quest narrative onto her life, MacGregor knows it has been closer to chaos.

Having absorbed various books and essays associated with the L'Arche movement, MacGregor notes that among others who write movingly of their encounters and experiences there, Henri J. M. Nouwen, rightly revered as a profound thinker on disability and Christian living, details stories that could be most clearly characterized as quest. MacGregor contrasts his and other thought-leaders' accounts with those of mothers like herself; the central difference is that these writers, as incisive as they are, have not experienced the relentless demands of lifelong caregiving:

> Nouwen [and others] chose to be caregivers, had opportunities to structure their caregiving responsibilities to accommodate their personal needs and abilities, and could cease caregiving when needed, or when desired. Their published narratives tell the preferred quest story because [they] had the means and power to limit the chaos often associated with chronic, complex caregiving.

These thoughts show me my own need for a redemptive narrative to shape both my and others' experiences. In some way, this is not wrong – as Christians, we *do* hope for the future; without this hope the universe would be the cold, empty void envisioned by Richard Dawkins, with no one there to hear our cries in the dark. We believe differently, but can we truly believe it without dismissing others' chaos stories as a lack of faith?

MacGregor clearly articulates that the lack of support from her faith community was one of her greatest disappointments. As a church, we need a vision of the kingdom of God so we can truly point toward God's unrelenting care and love for all people, including autistic people and their families.

Whether we stand in the church or the secular world, our faulty assumption, according to Brock, is the failure to acknowledge that all humanity is broken to some degree, and to perceive that people with intellectual disabilities are often able to exhibit kingdom patterns more powerfully than those who are neurotypical. My son says things precisely as he sees them – there is no hidden or cryptic meaning to decipher. Life is slower for many with intellectual disabilities and their families, and this model directly challenges the constant busyness and striving of modern life.

For Brock, the future converges with the present: his son Adam and others with autism are not subjects of speculation about what life will be like in heaven, or even primarily a conduit of the Spirit's gifts to the church, although they are that too. First and foremost, Adam is someone to be enjoyed, both by his parents and the church community:

> Such a hope expresses a . . . Spirit-gifted strength to love with the love that does not simply tolerate others but can say with unfeigned sincerity: "I'm glad you're here." This hope overlaps the paler belief that what "the disabled" bring to churches and individuals is a reminder of the dependence of every human being, or a sense of satisfaction of achieving inclusivity. Such a hope moves beyond the normal-disabled dichotomy in the prayer that our eyes will be opened to them, will see with eyes made to participate in a divine vision: "the Lord does not see as mortals see; they look on the outward appearance, but the Lord looks on the heart" (1 Sam. 16:7).

In the kingdom of God, his reign is unopposed. And his kingdom's manifestation here on earth sets us on a very different quest, not of fixing, or mending, or searching for tidy endings. No, it is harder; in the chaos of our own and others' lives, we must learn not to do, but to be. The good news for me, for the church, for that mother and her son, for everyone, is that God does not abandon us. He comes into our chaos; he walks with us as we learn to perceive his way.

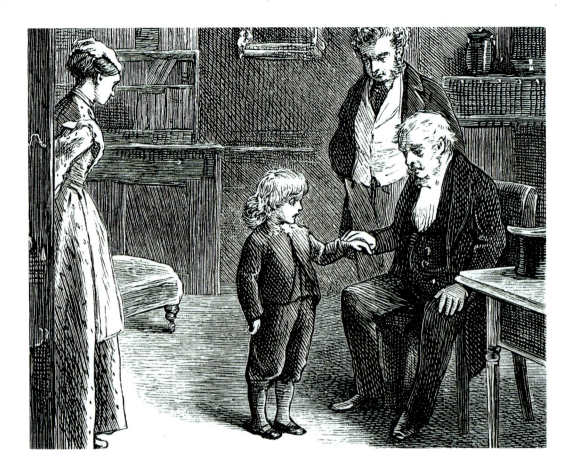

A Better Way to Doctor

The direct primary care model aims to put relationships over profit.

BREWER EBERLY

I DID NOT EXPECT to enjoy family medicine. My father and grandfather were both family doctors, yet when I started studying medicine myself, I was quick to discover a polite disrespect for primary care. "Why would you go into family medicine?" was a common refrain. This, despite a shortage of primary care doctors that is only expected to worsen.

The reasons have been rehearsed many times: the burden of documentation, the pressure to shorten patient encounters, the focus on metrics, the distractions of integrating third-party payers. The primary care doctors I met during medical school seemed the most jaded and world-weary. By the time I graduated, I was still proud of my family legacy but had written off a future in primary care.

Nineteenth-century illustration of a doctor paying a home visit to a young patient.

AROUND THE SAME TIME, a physician named Ben Fischer was growing dismayed by what he was encountering as an internist in an insurance-based primary care practice. He called it the "physician reprogramming project," in which he was being slowly malformed to focus more on quality improvement and financial throughput than on patient care, hurrying through his visits to check the bureaucracy's boxes, despite sensing in his heart that his patients were crying out for more. Ben began to wonder what a doctor is for beyond the efficient and effective participation in the health care industry. More deeply, Ben sensed he was not becoming the good doctor he had aspired to be.

Ben returned to a novel he already knew well, Wendell Berry's *Jayber Crow*, and found himself weeping. Jayber, the titular town barber, makes house calls to the farmer Athey Keith in the last months of his life, following a series of strokes, to cut his hair and be with him. Ben said to himself, "I want to doctor like Jayber barbered."

So Ben wrote to Wendell Berry. Berry wrote back, "I am always delighted to hear from professionally dissatisfied physicians." The Berrys invited Ben and his wife, Liz, to their farm in Kentucky, where they sat around their kitchen table and talked about how one might reform primary care. In 2016, the Fischers founded the clinic in which I now practice.

THE FISCHERS had already discovered the direct primary care movement before meeting with the Berrys. Since then, direct primary care (DPC) has become one of the fastest growing models in the United States, offering unlimited primary care for a periodic fee, without billing insurance. DPC's growth was driven in large part by primary care clinicians who had come to feel alienated from the patients they hoped to know and heal. By rejecting third-party involvement and redoubling attention to the doctor-patient relationship, the direct primary care doctor works solely for his or her patient for a flat fee, anywhere from $55 to $150 per month depending on the clinician.

In our practice, an average of $70 per month gives patients 24/7 access to their physician by phone and essentially limitless in-person visits. This monthly fee also covers simple in-office procedures and house calls. I recently visited two families with a dozen kids between them. It was a rowdy, intimate affair – requiring many paperclips and folders – but a gift to both me and these two families, who didn't have to think about scheduling separate well child checks across the year.

We even offer inpatient care, following our patients in the hospital, as their hospitalists, without charging extra. Patients still need "catastrophic" insurance to cover their actual stay, but they experience our presence in the hospital as a work of solidarity. As one of Ben's patients put it: "I found Dr. Fischer standing at the foot of my bed, waiting for me to wake up, just checking on me. . . . It made me feel very safe and cared for." I'll never forget seeing one of my own patients in the emergency room, where she said, "Thank you for coming. It has been so many strangers." I've learned that having "hospital privileges" does not just mean legal authorization to work in a hospital, but the actual *privilege* of caring for my patients in the home, clinic, and hospital.

Our practice is not necessarily representative of the larger DPC movement, which is variegated and decentralized, undergirded by different moral assumptions, political postures, and theological convictions. Still, direct primary care has given us something of a rescue boat, which we can fill with our love. We strive to practice according to our conviction that the health and wholeness of

---

Brewer Eberly is a third-generation family physician at Fischer Clinic in Raleigh, North Carolina, and a McDonald Agape Fellow in the Theology, Medicine, and Culture Initiative at Duke Divinity School.

our patients should be our sole work. We aim to know our patients well, know our profession well, and serve our patients directly in a way that offers them our attention, presence, and availability.

Because we do not bill insurance, we can link directly with nearby labs, pharmacies, and imaging centers to reduce costs. Together, the patient and physician can make practical, transparent, local decisions about what is best clinically and financially. We are able to serve patients pro bono if they can't pay, which is not always possible in traditional primary care settings because it would violate insurance contracts. To make this a reality, we partner with local ministries, employ sliding scales, and even barter. Many are the days my partners and I have been paid in sweet potatoes.

DIRECT PRIMARY CARE is a good example of subsidiarity, the principle that it is best to push responsibility to individuals and communities through local organization rather than relying on larger, more remote powers. It assumes that those who are closest to their neighbors know best what needs their neighbors have. As Catholic surgeon Donald Condit writes in *A Prescription for Health Care Reform*, "subsidiarity helps to ensure that love does not remain a vague gesture of goodwill toward all coupled with a failure to practice charity toward actual persons with whom we come in contact."

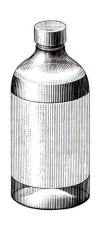
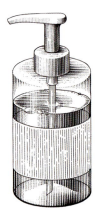

In many ways, modern primary care discourages subsidiarity. It prioritizes volume over relational depth. The average primary care doctor today takes care of something like 2,300 patients. But even following the reckoning of the health care industry, the number of patients a primary care doctor can actually accommodate per year within reasonable working hours is around 980. In the DPC model, however, such extrapolations are tempered by the actual experience of caring for suffering people, who often require time beyond what is clinically actionable. DPC physicians serve an average of 413 patients. I currently care for 604 people, some a few months old and some on the cusp of 100. The direct primary care patient receives over two hours of care per year compared to 33 minutes in traditional systems.

When patients sense their physician has structured a system that prioritizes relationship, other goods of solidarity emerge. In 2021, the *British Journal of General Practice* published a large study on continuity of care, based on 4.5 million people, which found that patients who had the same family doctor for just two years were 30 percent less likely to need to be admitted to the hospital and 25 percent less likely to *die* than those who had been with the same doctor less than a year. The likelihood of needing emergency care steadily dropped based on being known by your doctor.

In residency, getting calls in the middle of the night was difficult not because of interrupted sleep, but because I did not know my patient. It was clinically challenging to get a sense of the complexity of the story from which a stranger was calling out to me. I defaulted to CYA: "covering your ass." Frank speech felt impossible. I also found that misanthropic and dehumanizing humor festered when we did not know our patients personally.

The inverse is also true. Strong relationships breed candor. I recently sat with two patients, one of whom interrupted me suddenly and asked, "Why don't doctors talk to us normally? Like, why do you talk like a normal person?" I think her comment had less to do with me and more to do with this model, which cultivates honesty, and – blessedly – good humor. As a patient once told me, "I need you to be a shit screen." (I said, "Let me grab my white coat!")

Far from choosing an "easy" patient load, as I've been accused of by critics of DPC, we are choosing to be indefinitely on call, believing it is a critical feature of good medicine that a patient be able to see or speak with her doctor during her time of need. As the sociologist Charles L. Bosk writes in *Forgive and Remember: Managing Medical Failure*, "the time when medical students are around the most is the time in which they can do the least, just as the time when doctors can do the most is the time in which they are available the least." Availability peaks during medical training and goes downhill from there. We are trying to reverse that.

The difficulty is letting go of the pretense that we can always accept more patients. We need to name our limits, like a farmer who knows there are only so many cows he can care for well in a given plot.

Now, when I get calls from patients in the middle of the night, I feel a deep sense of privilege and a kind of delight precisely because I recognize my neighbor. I finally feel not just "on call" but called. As one of my patients said after calling me late one evening, "This is why I am letting you care for me."

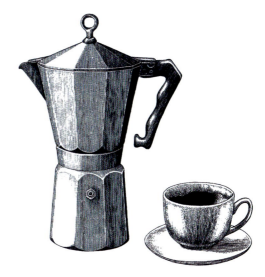

In his classic essay "To Be a Doctor," psychiatrist and medical historian Félix Martí-Ibáñez argues that "greatness is simplicity." The simplicity of DPC clears away distractions to focus on the care of patients. And yet I am well aware that how we do that still depends on what we believe and value. Our particular practice draws inspiration from Wendell Berry, but also physicians such as Leon Kass, Francis Peabody, and Farr Curlin, who seek to refocus the clinician's attention on health as the purpose of good medicine. As Curlin puts it, we are seeking "just medicine, for those who need it." And ultimately, our work is not separated from our friendships and shared faith as three physicians who look to Christ as our hope and stay. While we do not make these "radical sources" apparent to our patients, they infuse all we do.

But I'll confess, after three years of practicing in this place that I deeply love, alongside physicians and nurses I profoundly respect and admire, I still have lingering questions. Because we are no longer linked up with "the system," I sometimes struggle to offer the care I aspire to. For example, it is often difficult to sustain long-term relationships with our most vulnerable patients. Disparities manifest in everything from mistrust to housing instability to a lack of transportation, making it difficult for us to maintain continuity. As one academic direct primary care practice found, despite launching with the explicit purpose of serving low-income and uninsured patients, "effective partnerships are crucial and elusive." Tellingly, the practice closed because it could not sustain the volume necessary to support itself.

There are other critiques of DPC practices. For one, they are not required to participate in HIPAA or HITECH. Theoretically, they have less oversight because they are not obligated to participate in quality measurement programs or shared

Summer 2025 75

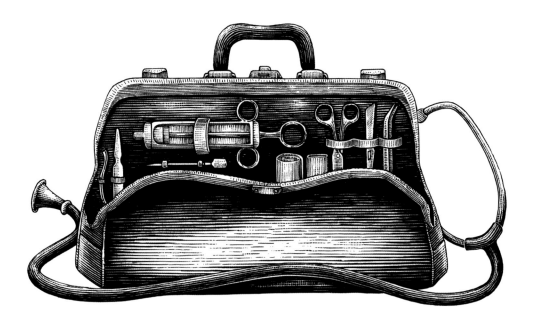

electronic health records, which could reveal problems with coordination of care, guideline adherence, or malpractice. In DPC's defense, there are ongoing open studies to address this, such as the "Direct Primary Care Medical Malpractice Audit and Program Feasibility Study," but these depend on the transparency of individual DPC physicians willing to submit information.

On the other hand, it is difficult for general physicians to hide unworthy work when they have intentionally embedded themselves in the community they serve. We are not rogue clinical cowboys; we've taken the same oaths and are held to the same professional standards. Our "quality measurement program" is our reputation in the community and among our clinical colleagues.

DPC is often conflated with, and dismissed as, "concierge medicine." While concierge medicine developed alongside DPC in the 1990s, concierge practices usually charge a retainer on top of billing insurance, so are generally an option only for those who can afford "double charging." DPC is not concierge, but the perception is hard to shake.

Most DPC practices do not interact with Medicare and Medicaid and therefore risk a lack of attention to the poor and elderly, leading to charges that DPC primarily serves the "healthy wealthy." Then there is the awkwardness of exchanging money directly with patients who are your neighbors. I believe our model is just, but as bioethicist M. Therese Lysaught points out, Christians did not begin caring for the sick under a grammar of disposable wealth or "philanthropy attached to a profitable enterprise," but with a love that transformed political and social arrangements into something new. Examples of this today include the Christ House for the homeless, the "money-free medicine" of the Bruderhof, and the Hawthorne Dominicans, who care for those with incurable cancer. Wendell Berry writes, "Work done in gratitude, kindly and well, is prayer. This is not for hire. You make yourself a way for love to reach the ground." I long to work purely for love, but I am, in fact, for hire – *paid* to care.

At the same time, I think of how the ability of Christian bishops in the fourth century to offer hospice depended on the charity of wealthy Christians. I've wondered if I should have joined an FQHC (Federally Qualified Health Center) or some other "safety net" system to avoid this tension, but even in such places I've encountered primary care physicians who burned out because they replaced maximum production of insured patients with maximum production of impoverished patients. As a former FQHC clinician put it to me, they still often "follow corporate empire logic."

A revealing cautionary tale is the Medicaid-managed direct primary care practice Qliance, founded in 2007 in Seattle as the nation's largest DPC health care system, serving thirty-five thousand patients, half of whom were covered by Medicaid. Beguiled by political and investor pressures, Qliance filed for bankruptcy in 2018, despite showing early promise.

Direct primary care is, I'm convinced, less dehumanizing for doctors than other models. At the same time, I see in the movement a self-assurance that risks missing the work of reform left to be done. DPC physicians can find themselves attacking health care as business while becoming successful business people.

When my grandfather was a family physician, he wrote that we need young doctors of "integrity, energy, and charity." It has proven far harder than I imagined to build a practice that sustains the physician's integrity, restores the burnt-out doctor to energy, and cultivates charity.

Haggard generalists may be choosing direct primary care because they think it will make medicine easier. Direct primary care hasn't made my work easier, though it has made it more serious, joyful, clear, and close. It has removed anonymity and the miasma of bureaucratic task-mastering, which can insidiously wear one down to the point of burnout, chronic moral injury, or resignation.

I have found that since I left "the system," my awareness of my own failings has become more acute. Now, on days when I am frustrated, angry, or inattentive, I can no longer blame "the system." It is, in fact, my heart that still needs to change, and my own clinical acumen that still needs sharpening. I am brought into a naked confrontation with my own lack of spiritual gifts. To riff on C. S. Lewis in *Out of the Silent Planet*, I find myself "an agent as well as a patient." I strive for my work to be healing to patients, but it has been an unexpected gift to find myself healing too.

Direct primary care is not a panacea; it is a platform. Its success will depend on the character of the practitioners it enables and the local communities surrounding them. Freedom does not guarantee one will use that freedom well. As Erika Bliss, the mother of direct primary care, once quipped, patients looking to direct primary care must discern between those doctors running *from* something and those running *to* something.

In our practice, we are candid with patients. We are not just running from a broken system but running toward relationship. We are not a fine-dining restaurant but a local diner, in which you are not the only patron, but in which you can expect recognition, hospitality, and a good meal. You won't get the luxury of having a private doctor in your pocket but rather the gift of having a doctor in the family, who can be reached when you are in need, without fighting a phone tree.

When Ben Fischer met with Wendell Berry, one of the first things Berry did was connect him to another local physician to discern together the rough path ahead. We remain deeply in need of our friends from other specialties and health care disciplines, along with our pastors and of course our patients, to hold us accountable to the good work we are setting out to do.

Take away the powers and principalities of modern medicine; reify the aims and double down on fidelity; and you are still left with the human heart, struggling to find the real work. Whatever the framework, we doctors are still left with the sick who come to us hoping for healing, until the fever of life is over and our work is done. As one of my first patients told me, "I look forward to dying with you." That feels like a call to doctor the way Jayber barbered.

REVIEWS

Editors' Picks

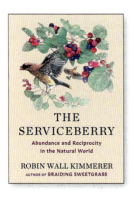

The Serviceberry

Robin Wall Kimmerer

(Scribner, 128 pages)

The Serviceberry is a short book with a heavy burden. Robin Wall Kimmerer, a distinguished environmental biology professor and a member of the Citizen Potawatomi Nation, has been out under the serviceberry trees, thinking about what is wrong with the global economic system. The mixed market economies in which most of us live, she argues, have reduced us to self-interested, greedy competitors, imprisoned in "patterns of gross overconsumption that have brought us to the brink of disaster." In the serviceberry economy, though, Kimmerer sees only generosity and abundance: gifts of carbon dioxide and solar waves to the serviceberry, gifts of sugar to the pollinating flies and cedar waxwings, gifts of feathers to the beetles, who are themselves gifts to the voles, whose carcasses feed the microorganisms, who build the soil, which in turn nourishes the serviceberry. Out here, she writes, "all flourishing is mutual." It could be so with humans, says Kimmerer, as suggested by alternative economic arrangements such as Indigenous potlatches, little free libraries, open-source software projects, and – in what seems to be the genesis of the essay – the sharing of serviceberries by her farmer neighbors. Gift economies abound in the world's unnoticed corners.

The targets of Kimmerer's ire are massive global forces – governments, corporations, and systemic greed – while her heroes are mostly neighbors and friends. The contrast is too glib, and it sidesteps the question of whether gift economies can *only* exist in the shadow or ruins of such large-scale systems. The little free library books were printed by cutthroat publishing companies. The "free knowledge" available on YouTube and TikTok is heavily monetized. Looking to the natural world for models of moral economy is perilous, whether it is the grim winner-takes-all vision that Kimmerer critiques, or the harmonious mutualism that she cheers. On a planet where some 40 percent of all animal species are parasites, where eating means that someone else dies, all flourishing is mutual only if our definition of "flourishing" includes piracy, cannibalism, and countless painful deaths. The world may be stunningly beautiful, as Annie Dillard underscored in *Pilgrim at Tinker Creek*, but it is also "festering with suppurating sores."

Kimmerer's vision – full of sweet-tart berries, chortling birds, and the Indigenous tradition of the "Honorable Harvest" – is a sunnier version of the "possibility of life in capitalist ruins" in Anna Lowenhaupt Tsing's *The Mushroom at the End of the World*, or the strangely hopeful rewilding of the world's "eeriest and most desolate places" in Cal Flyn's *Islands of Abandonment*. We certainly need hope, and we need to see the gifts we have been given, especially in a twenty-first-century economy where companies seem pleased to help us transform every part of our lives into income-producing assets: spare rooms into hotels, extra seats into taxis, and our looks, families, hobbies, and aesthetic tastes into "personal brands." And on this point Kimmerer is right: it need not be so. The Israelites lived for decades on a mysterious bread that fell from the sky each morning with the dew. Jesus commended the economic attitudes of sparrows and lilies and satisfied five thousand people with a single meager meal.

—*William Thomas Okie*

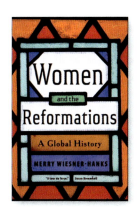

Women and the Reformations
A Global History

Merry Wiesner-Hanks

(Yale University Press, 364 pages)

"If they were to burn me tomorrow or drown me in a sack, that's all the same to me," said Weynken Claes, thought to be the first female Protestant martyr, before being burned at the stake in The Hague in 1527. Englishwoman Anne Line showed similar courage in 1601 by stating, in her trial for harboring Catholic priests, that she wished "that where I had entertained one, I could have entertained a thousand." She would lose her life on the gallows. The stories of these women and dozens of others appear in Merry Wiesner-Hanks's *Women and the Reformations*.

Although not the first book written on Reformation-era women, its variety of sources and stories sets it apart. Grouped thematically as monarchs, mothers, migrants, martyrs, mystics, and missionaries, narratives of Protestant, Catholic, Anabaptist, Jewish, and Muslim women are juxtaposed in a complex tapestry that blurs confessional boundaries. Wiesner-Hanks draws attention to how women's experiences differed from men's – sometimes exceptions were made for women; more often, they fell under greater scrutiny. But she also shows how these women's commitment to their convictions about how God ought to be worshiped sustained them in acts of astonishing resistance.

The chapter on monarchs shows that women were often influential in the religious world: the first rulers to grant religious tolerance in their domains were queens. The following chapter, "Mothers," is a goldmine of cultural history, profiling women of low social status alongside nuns and the wives of reformers. The featured migrants come from varied backgrounds: Anabaptist Katharina Hutter, Jewish and Muslim women expelled from Spain, and the Spanish nuns who helped missionize Japan. Mystics – from Spain to Peru, England to the Congo – seem to have ended up either disgraced or canonized. Throughout, stories from regions outside of Europe stretch the reader's understanding of the wide impact of the Reformation – or, more accurately, reformations.

Although this era's histories have generally highlighted canonical male leaders, this book points to a far more complex reality. Writing as a historian, Wiesner-Hanks includes women whose lives and thought do not fit easily into the molds of orthodoxy – some even veering into the heretical. Although straightforward hagiographies have their place, nuanced narratives that show both the flaws of heroines and the tenacity of heretics can inform the reader's own search.

All the women featured in this book suffered, some horrendously. But Wiesner-Hanks includes humorous moments too. Nuns resisting the Lutheranization of their convents stuffed wax in their ears or sang during sermons and even ignited old felt slippers to drive the preacher out with the resulting putrid smoke. Jansenist sisters in northern France dodged a summons to sign an oath of adherence to Catholic orthodoxy by claiming that women were biblically barred from opining on theological matters. The bones of Catherine Dammartin, a former nun who married the Italian reformer Peter Vermigli, were combined with those of Saint Frideswide to keep both Protestants and Catholics from desecrating the dead.

Though the violence done to these women is appalling, their zeal and steadfastness is admirable. This book reads as a call to ecumenism, encouraging a greater appreciation for the way women view and live out their relationship to God.

—*Coretta Thomson*

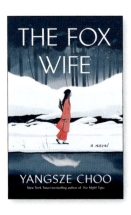

The Fox Wife
A Novel

Yangsze Choo

(Holt Paperbacks, 400 pages)

In one story, a fox spirit seeks revenge. The spirit, named Snow, takes the form of a beautiful woman or an otherworldly white fox. She, like all fox spirits, can beguile and seduce humans, but is also vulnerable to human suspicion and physical strength. Despite the danger, the heartbroken Snow ventures into the city to take her revenge on the man who killed her daughter.

In the other story, a sixty-three-year-old detective named Bao is hired to solve the murder of a woman. He is observant, kind, and shrewd, even as his aging body has begun to fail him. Bao has been fascinated by stories of fox spirits since he was a boy, but he shoves his belief to the side, no longer hoping for such a magical world. Still, his case continues to bring up rumors of foxes, and soon he begins to wonder if he is on a fox's trail.

Yangsze Choo's *The Fox Wife* is a delightful blend of genres set at the turn of the twentieth century in Manchuria, Mongolia, and Japan. Bao's tale is a classic detective story, with flashbacks that blend coming-of-age with romance. *The Fox Wife* is part fairy story, part revenge thriller, and part comedy of manners as Snow takes on the role of a household servant (fox schemes, as it turns out, often involve a lot of unexpected complications and improvisation). The novel's refusal to settle into one genre is fitting, since, as Snow relates to her readers, "the mark of a fox is to disrupt order." And, as it turns out, there is more than one fox in this story.

Although Snow's story originates in a great tragedy, Choo's novel does not wallow in darkness. Its playful sense of humor is demonstrated when Snow relates fox-facts such as, "Foxes are incurably nosy. That's why you'll often find us at festivals, riots, and other people's birthday parties." There is also a sense of something other, something that refuses to settle in light or dark, just beneath the surface of Snow's quest for vengeance and Bao's pursuit of a killer. This is the nature of a fairy story – or here, of a fox story – since "Humans and things are different species, and foxes lie between humans and things; darkness and light take different paths, and foxes lie in between darkness and light."

Snow is aware that the magic of foxes is fading in the face of modernity. Hiding and living in the margins is becoming more difficult in a world of rapid population growth, train travel, and photography. Bao, meanwhile, knows he has lost something essential when he grew beyond his "childish" hope to meet a fox one day. He "can't quite bring himself to embrace such superstition, yet neither can he abandon it. At the edge of his raging curiosity lurks the possibility of the divine, an unknown veil that Bao longs to pierce." This is where *The Fox Wife*'s excellence lies: in Choo's insight into the longing for enchantment – and in her ability to tell an entertaining, wily, and unpredictable tale.

—*James Smoker*

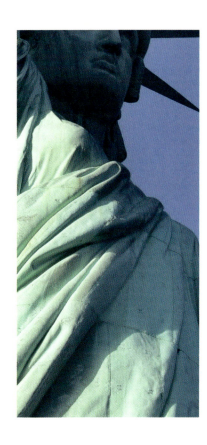

On the Staten Island Ferry

As we pull away from the pier
the bundled variegated crowd
of commuters and tourists, pilgrims of a kind,
chattering in a medley of mother tongues,
flock to starboard
e pluribus unum
to catch a glimpse as we pass.
I realize I've never seen
Liberty in person, lifting up her lamp—
a celebrity in the flesh,
although her flesh is copper, her bones iron
(a cousin to Monsieur Eiffel's *dame de fer*)
and though the golden door in days like these
is shut against the yearnings of the huddled masses and the poor
she stands there, great with gravitas, clothed in verdigris
(the "green of Greece," she is an ancient goddess!)
colossal yet a woman, dwarfed by sky-crowding towers.
And then I hear the black-haired girl in a pink coat, who points
tugging at her mother's sleeve,
hopping in a little joyful dance.
"*Mira!* There she is!
She's beautiful!"
(Her mother adds, she was a gift from France.)
"She's beautiful," says the girl, "even though she's green!
She's beautiful, even though she isn't real!"
And we all lean
out for a better look
and I'm surprised by everything I feel.

A. E. STALLINGS

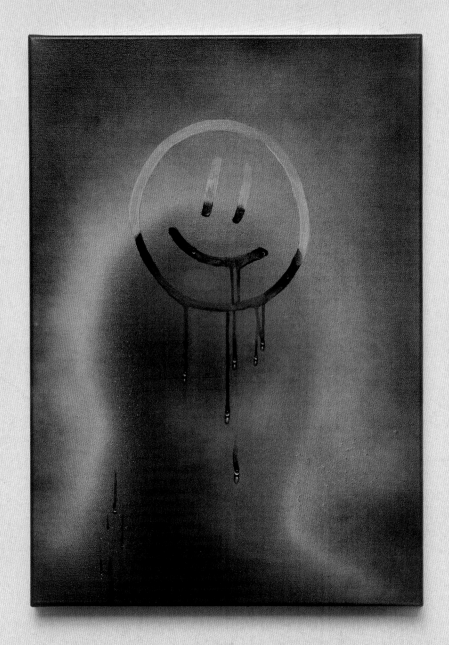

Desire, Use, Repeat

An addict looks for a way out.

JAMES MUMFORD

I'VE BEEN IN A TWELVE-STEP PROGRAM, or, as they (I mean we) say, "recovery," for about five minutes. So, I'm obviously ready to make an authoritative set of observations.

I had never drunk vodka for breakfast. Nor injected heroin between my toes. I clung to those horror stories when I first came into "the rooms" (the preferred nomenclature for twelve-step meetings). Why? Dwelling on that species of "rock bottom" helped me deny the fact that my name is James and I'm an addict.

I am addicted to everything, or at least everything I can get my hands on. Nicotine. Alcohol. Caffeine. Prescription meds. Food. Sex. Spending. It doesn't matter what the substance is. Sugar is porn! My drug of choice is more. My story, as American novelist and essayist Leslie Jamison writes of her own, comes down "to the same demolished and reductive and recycled core: Desire. Use. Repeat."

IN THE WAKE OF MY SEPARATION and divorce, I found a highly respectable, sympathetic drug dealer within the discreetly brass-plated Harley Street drug-den that is my beloved private doctor's office.

I needed this because the local NHS clinic in East London had let me down. They had refused to prescribe me Zopiclone and Valium. I needed that medicine, I insisted, to regulate sleep and manage anxiety. That's what I told them. That's what I told myself. But shortsighted and resource strapped as socialized medicine is, the NHS wasn't having any of it.

Easier to manipulate was my tall, languid, private doctor in his Henry Poole double-breasted suit with his double-barreled name. He was a far cry from Tuco Salamanca, the short, psychotic, gold-toothed drug kingpin in *Breaking Bad*. My man was charming and obliging and seemed to have all the time in the world for me. The leisurely appointments were a delight! We got on famously, breezily discussing all manner of topics. (Why is the Unites States so polarized? Which is the best independent school in London?) I wouldn't be having these kinds of conversations with this kind of person if my life were falling apart, if I were the kind of person whose life could fall apart. My new confidante – I counted him a friend, really – was willing to listen for hour upon billable hour.

In truth, I wanted the drugs to cut out the long, lonely evenings now that my routine was no longer reading *The Voyage of the Dawn Treader* to my daughters before cajoling or bribing them to brush their teeth (molars included, get that toothbrush all the way in the back). I used to wish I had more time to read. Now I have all the time in the world to read. So, drugs were the way I could slink away from the world – earlier and earlier in the day. Like Romeo sequestered in his bedroom, I'd shut up my windows, lock fair light out, and make myself an artificial night. Drugs were the way I'd try to quash the pain. *Desire, use, repeat.* The euphoria you get before passing out with Zopiclone, like the courtesan's final energetic aria in *La Traviata* before she succumbs to her tuberculosis, allowed me to change the way I felt. "By feigned deaths to die" is how John Donne describes such prolonged absences. The more straightforward way to put it is that drugs were the means by which I could fuck off for a bit.

Apart from my man in Harley Street, no one knew about this. I hadn't let anyone else in. Why would I? So my friends could dissuade me? But I'd resolved on this way of coping. No one

---

James Mumford is an English writer, the author of Vexed: Ethics Beyond Political Tribes *(Bloomsbury, 2020) and* Therapized: How Psychology Hurts the People It's Meant to Help *(Little Brown, 2026).*

Opposite: Jochen Mühlenbrink, *JMWP Smile*, oil and acrylics on canvas, 2024.

knowing, however, meant no one identifying the increasing regularity with which I got high. It meant no one could warn me. Soon the odd treat was not enough. I started taking Zopiclone daily, and when I acclimated, taking more,

---

The therapy-speak that has become common, with its blanket affirmation of "my truth" as opposed to "the truth," often facilitates denial of my own part in sowing the chaos I'm reaping.

---

upping the dosage, then supplementing it with Valium. After all, not being able to sleep while addicted to sleeping pills is anxiety-inducing! In the end, every night I risked slipping into a coma. Anything to avoid lying on my side on my bed, forced to relive and re-narrate the last months of my marriage – those things I ought to have done, those things I ought not to have done.

TWELVE-STEP FELLOWSHIPS famously pride themselves on being spiritual, not religious. The act of surrender so critical to overcoming addiction (we "made a decision to turn our will and our lives over . . . ," according to step 2) is to be made to a "higher power" or "God as we understood Him." Despite this, what strikes me as a newcomer is how liturgical AA is. For someone hailing from a charismatic-evangelical background with no set liturgy or unison prayers or spoken creeds, AA seems remarkably high church.

Take the structure of your average AA meeting. It commences with creedal proclamation; tattered, laminated cards are read out – "The Twelve Steps," "Twelve Traditions," or "The Promises" – as well as a daily reflection and an extract from the semi-sacred text that is "the Big Book." Then there's a testimony or "chair": an invited speaker – sometimes a regular, sometimes a guest – shares their "experience, strength, and hope" for fifteen minutes. Next is communal confession: for a carefully timed three minutes people "share back" to the speaker (but not, crucially, to each other; this counts as "crosstalk" and is discouraged so what you say won't be publicly criticized). Typically, people vocalize what resonates with them in the story they've just heard ("look for the similarity, not the differences") or else they open up ("honesty in meetings helps us to stay sober") about what it's like climbing back from the eighth circle of hell. Then comes the sacrament (different colored chips handed out for recovery milestones) and a kind of altar call (a chip for anyone who wants to commit to a new way of life). The meeting then closes with corporate petition (the "Serenity Prayer" written by the midcentury American neoorthodox theologian Reinhold Niebuhr). *God, grant me the serenity to accept the things I cannot change, the courage to change the things I can, and the wisdom to know the difference.*

It's not just that the meetings are liturgical; AA also revolves around a rule of life. The Twelve Steps are introduced in the literature as "a group of principles, spiritual in nature, which, if practiced as a way of life, can expel the obsession to drink and enable the sufferer to become happily and usefully whole." It is a way of life because it is a daily program. Only by focusing relentlessly on the day, hour, minute at hand, only by refusing to wander around in the past and future ("times that do not belong to us," as Pascal wrote), can one hope to overcome addiction. Liberation hinges on taking a positively monastic approach to living.

IN OUR CULTURE, most problems are construed as general, the solutions specific. Someone says he suffers from anxiety; one friend recommends Hatha Yoga to solve this problem; a second suggests walks in nature, a third medication. AA reverses this. The problem is specific: alcoholics can't stop drinking when everyone else

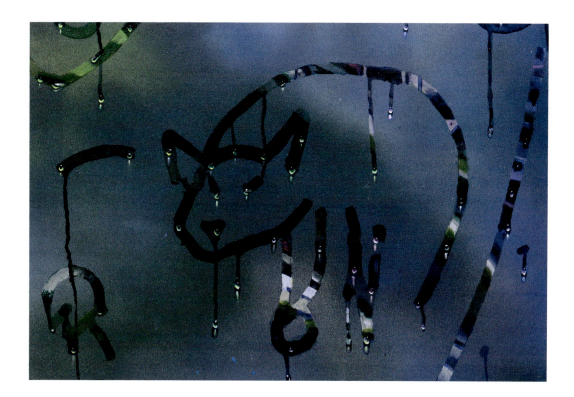

does. But then the solution is general: *becoming a better person.*

If you'd asked me what people talk about in an AA meeting before I'd attended my first one, I would've guessed they sat around discussing their favorite gin substitutes. In fact, what fellows talk about is wanting to live a life worthy of a human being. They talk about what they have done, or what they are realizing they need to do – the action they need to take – to be able to live with themselves: actions like risking the truth at work; showing up as a parent; or regaining the trust of their spouse. They talk, that is, about learning to be good.

This is the reason why recovery is such a potent antidote to our therapized culture. This may not be true of all therapy, but the therapeutic intervention I experienced as a patient in a psychiatric hospital I found profoundly de*moral*izing. Being told by a psychologist that "values are subjective" made me feel worse, and left me more depressed.

Why? Because in the grip of depression, the only things I knew to be true about the world were certain orienting convictions about right and wrong – that abuse is always wicked, and goodness not merely a matter of perspective. But these were convictions my psychologist was inadvertently contesting when he – with all the authority of his credentials – informed me that morality is merely "externally imposed by society." He was taking a sledgehammer to my moral compass; I was left reeling, bereft of coordinates, consigned to the position of those the psalmist speaks about: "There be many that say, Who will shew us any good?" (Psalm 4:6).

The twelve-step outlook is radically different: it avoids the pitfall of indulgence as well as that of judgmentalism. The therapy-speak that has become common in the workplace and the family, with its blanket affirmation of "my truth" as opposed to "the truth," all too often facilitates denial of my own part in sowing the chaos I'm

Jochen Mühlenbrink, *NYWP* (detail), oil and acrylics on canvas.

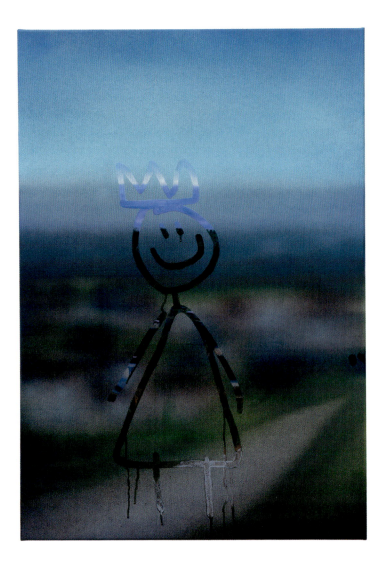

person-centered therapists insist upon "unconditional positive regard." But in recovery, while there's certainly a strong belief in the irreplaceable value of persons, we're also told that, in order to survive – let alone thrive – there are some things about oneself it makes sense *not* to accept. I wouldn't, frankly, wish my authentic self on my worst enemy. Instead, we are instructed, kindly but firmly, to find the "courage to change the things we can." The idea of making "a searching and fearless moral inventory of ourselves" (step 4), admitting "the exact nature of our wrongs" (step 5), and then being willing to consent to the removal of "all these defects of character" (step 6), would be anathema to many psychoanalysts; it might even be deemed abusive.

reaping in my own life and in the lives of others. Say I've come to identify greed or lust or pride in myself; my therapist assures me that we are all in the same boat; that there's nothing to be done; and that these should not be thought of as vices to be repented of but as, perhaps, coping strategies to be understood. Twelve-step recovery is readier to recognize that some boats are sinking, and that honor among thieves is scant consolation when the dark waters begin to flood the deck.

Following Carl Rogers, the twentieth-century pioneer of humanistic psychology,

It is not. The twelve-step programs are bulwarks against nihilism, and their steady and consistent success among men and women of all kinds and conditions testifies to the match between what philosophers name "moral realism" – the insistence that some ways to live really are better than others – and achieving a flourishing life.

To PATHOLOGIZE is typically to exculpate; in other words, we don't blame people for being *ill*. Twelve-step fellowships, however, contest the assumption that the specific disease

Jochen Mühlenbrink, *WP Princess*, oil and acrylics on canvas, 2024.

that is addiction is exempt from moral evaluation. "We have come to believe [alcoholism] an illness," the Big Book reads, but an illness that "involves those about us in a way no other human sickness can." The collateral damage from addiction – at this juncture the Big Book lists "fierce resentment," "financial insecurity," "sad" spouses and the cost to children – can be immense, but it wasn't inevitable. AA is not heavily moralistic, but neither is it deterministic. It refuses to dissolve responsibility in the acid of fatalism. There may be strong genetic predispositions to addiction. There may be horrendous circumstances that precipitate it. There also remain choices. As an addict, one is unwell. But with this particular kind of sickness, one may learn to be well.

Surrender, too, is a choice. But what kind of choice? Does surrender to God entail an extinction of self, as many gurus insist – that is, an elimination of the desires that make up me?

At first it seems that a negation of desire is exactly what AA has in mind. "The only condition for membership is a desire to stop drinking," states the preamble read out at the beginning of every meeting. But in my experience desire is a moving target. What I want deep down at 7:30 a.m., fully caffeinated and ensconced in my morning AA meeting, is not always what I want at 7:30 p.m. when I'm hangry and my concentration is shot. And precisely because desire *wanes*, I am finding that perhaps a better bet than merely *desisting* from using (i.e., sitting on my hands, "white-knuckling it," trying to *stop wanting* to finagle drugs from a doctor) is, instead, to put myself in a position where I can be enticed by goods worthier of my attention. Indeed, in Saint Paul's ethical injunctions to the Ephesians, he doesn't simply counsel abstaining from vice but enumerates replacement activities:

> Let the thief no longer steal, but instead let him work, accomplishing something good with his own hands so that he might have it to share with the person in need. Out of your foul mouth let no utterance proceed, but instead whatever is good for needed edification, that it might impart a grace to those listening. (Eph. 4:28–29)

AA suggests a whole load of things to get on with. Sobriety is about taking up, not just giving up. So I am rediscovering long-forsaken hobbies; I'm listening to Counting Crows ballads circa 1993 on repeat; I'm studiously rewatching Alan Partridge sitcoms; I might even try to play for England again. I am attempting – for instance, by

---

I can't yet see all the good there is in this new health, but I have a hint. I have the end of a thread.

---

making calls to fellows in the old-fashioned hope of connection – to put myself in a position where I can be bewitched by alternative "objects" of attention, rival and more worthy objects of love. I can't yet see all the good there is in this new health, but I have a hint. I have the end of a thread. To follow that hint is to enter into all the life that lies in store, a life that I will, I must, show up for.

Perhaps this is what Iris Murdoch meant when she said we "grow by looking." Maybe she meant putting yourself in a position where you can at least get an unobstructed view of things you intuit to be more wholesome than those which preoccupy you now. Perhaps "growing by looking" is simply making yourself available for seizure, for an arrest that will ensure the radical reshaping of your desires.

Perhaps, finally, the search for the higher power who is the *Deus absconditus,* the hidden God, is like this too. Maybe I just have to shift my stance, as it were, or crane my neck round, so I can look in his general direction, this God of my understanding whom I know I cannot fully understand.

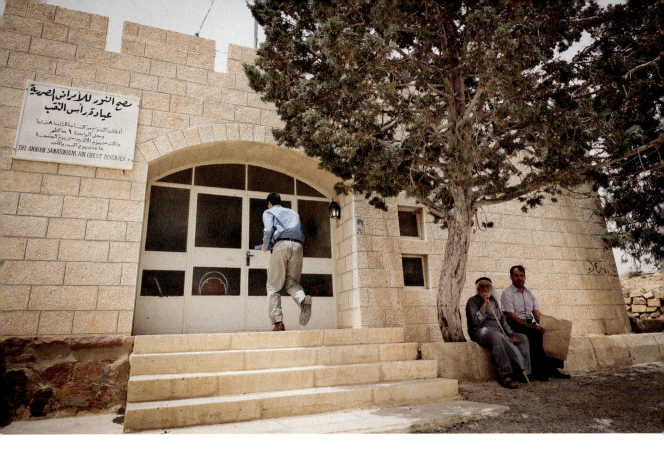

Healing at Annoor

A hospital in Mafraq, Jordan, serves patients with tuberculosis.

HEATHER M. SURLS

On Friday mornings, the city of Mafraq sleeps. It's the first day of the weekend in Jordan; midday, men and boys will trickle to local mosques for prayer before returning home for lunch with their families. Usually, downtown's grid of narrow, dusty streets is packed with honking traffic. This morning, shops are shuttered and cars parked.

For Laith Sahawneh, clinic manager at Annoor Sanatorium, Friday mornings are anything but quiet. In his office outside of central Mafraq, the landline rings. Text messages ping through his mobile phone. Pharmacists, doctors, and even patients pop in and out of his office, asking questions, seeking advice. Though it's the weekend, the hospital for chest diseases is open for business, accommodating patients who work a normal Sunday-through-Thursday week.

"We want to serve as many patients as we can," says Sahawneh, a Jordanian Christian.

With six exam rooms, a lab, and a pharmacy, Sahawneh tells me, clinic staff presently treat

Annoor Sanatorium's administrative building.

an average of two hundred outpatients per week. Before the Covid-19 pandemic, when Annoor established a phone-scheduling system to minimize crowding, admissions were more hectic. Sometimes more than one hundred sick people lined up at the hospital's gate before dawn, Sahawneh recalls.

Patients come to Annoor – which means "the light" in Arabic – with chronic chest illnesses: asthma, pulmonary fibrosis, brucellosis, tuberculosis. They come from all over Jordan – and even from other Arab countries, like Iraq, Saudi Arabia, and Yemen – attracted by the hospital's reputation. Annoor's doctors ask questions and listen to medical histories; they listen, rather than hurriedly diagnosing and prescribing. The staff treats their patients kindly, with love. Muslim patients accept prayers from their Christian doctors. Healing can be found at Annoor.

Sahawneh says that most of Annoor's patients have visited multiple doctors already, without seeing improvement. Because of this, 90 percent of the cases that come through the clinic are very difficult to treat. Some of the worst are admitted to Annoor's inpatient program, which hosts an average of fifteen at any given time. Most of these suffer from tuberculosis (TB), a bacterial disease that ravages the patient's lungs "like a terrorist, bombing and fighting," Sahawneh says. The disease, which in 2022 infected about four in 100,000 people in Jordan, can be treated through a strict regimen of several antibiotics taken over the course of six months.

Multidrug-resistant TB cases are even more difficult, some baffling the medical team – currently a group of six physicians from Egypt, Korea, the United States, and Britain. At times, healing seems preposterous from a human perspective. But miracles happen at Annoor – not magic, as some patients speculate. God intervenes on behalf of the sick, Sahawneh says, sometimes without the use of medicine.

"When you hear a request from the locals or the patients, you will say, 'This is impossible, how can I do it?'" he says. "Then, in a miraculous way, the Lord opens a path."

NEAR THE MEN'S WARD, a hallway leads to Nasri Khoury's office. Stacked with boxes and unused medical equipment, it resembles a storage area. In the smaller anteroom, chairs circle a table packed with cups and saucers and plastic containers of coffee and sugar. Photographs of Jordan's royal family and Annoor's founders decorate the walls. A stack of Bibles is piled on one chair.

Khoury – better known as Abu Steve, after his oldest son – has witnessed God's miraculous ways at Annoor since 1965, when the hospital opened in a 2,100-square-foot building in Mafraq. The town's population was less than seven thousand then, with five cars and five televisions. "I counted them," he says, a big smile on his face.

Khoury tells me about the hospital's early years as he prepares coffee over a tiny burner fueled by isopropyl alcohol. Herb Klassen, Annoor's executive director, later tells me that over thirty-five years of informal gatherings with male inpatients, Khoury has perfected the art of sharing the story of God's love in the time it takes to make coffee.

While he is Christian and most of his patients are Muslim, Khoury sees God's love as transcending those distinctions. "The angel came to tell us about a Savior, not Christianity," he says. "We are here to give the Good News."

Khoury grew up in Beit Sahour, a Palestinian Christian village near Bethlehem, and studied nursing at Baraka Hospital for Chest Diseases in

---

Heather M. Surls' reporting has appeared in Christianity Today *and* Religion News Service, *and her creative nonfiction in* Brevity *and* Ekstasis. *Her memoir-in-essays,* Beyond the Jordan, *releases from Lucid Books this summer. She lives in Amman, Jordan, with her husband and two sons.*

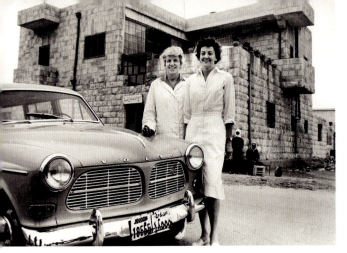

Arroub, south of Bethlehem. There he met Aileen Coleman, an Australian nurse and midwife, and Eleanor Soltau, an American thoracic physician. Both single women felt called by God to serve the Bedouin, who often do not recover fully from TB because of poverty and their nomadic lifestyle.

When theological differences with Baraka's leadership forced Coleman and Soltau to leave the hospital, they told Khoury they planned to one day start a TB hospital in Jordan and hoped that he would join them.

Shortly afterward, Coleman met Lester Gates in Jerusalem. A recently widowed farmer from Ohio, Gates was looking to start the next chapter in his life. He was inspired by Coleman's vision for the hospital and came to Jordan to help get it off the ground. Initially intending to come for six months, Gates ended up staying for twenty-two years, building Annoor with his own hands and financial resources.

In the meantime, Khoury took a profitable job at a hospital in Saudi Arabia. When Coleman and Soltau informed him they had returned to the Middle East, he requested a month of vacation to travel to Mafraq. His employer acquiesced, but also purchased Khoury's return ticket and refurnished his apartment on the Saudi hospital's compound.

A few weeks later, Khoury knelt in his room at Annoor with Gates, who would soon become his spiritual mentor. Together they sought God's will for Khoury's future: return to Saudi Arabia, or stay at Annoor, where his monthly salary was just eighteen Jordanian dinar. God's presence unmistakably filled the room, Khoury says, assuring him of God's direction.

"I took the plane ticket and burned it," he says.

By the late 1960s, Annoor needed a larger facility. Gates and Khoury borrowed the hospital's vehicle and drove until they found the piece of land that God had shown Gates in a dream: twenty-five bare acres just outside of Mafraq. When they asked Annoor's gate guard about the land, he informed them that it belonged to Mafraq's mayor.

Khoury felt reluctant to approach the mayor: What right had he, a young nurse, to ask the community's leader to sell his land? But the next day, when Khoury explained that Annoor was hoping to purchase a piece of land for a new facility, he didn't even have to ask.

"I have one," the mayor volunteered.

Annoor acquired the land for just two thousand dollars. Right away, Khoury says, Gates started planting trees like crazy – eight thousand pine trees donated by the Jordanian Ministry of Agriculture, hundreds of olive and fruit trees. "The more trees we plant, the more souls will come to the Lord," Gates reasoned.

When the government insisted they would not find water on the property, Gates insisted otherwise. They drilled on the spot God showed him and hit water. Since 1973, when Annoor moved to its permanent location, the hospital has operated on water from its own well.

"It's so beautiful to walk in God's ways," Khoury reflects. "When we walk in God's ways, he arranges everything."

NOW NINETY-FOUR YEARS OLD, Coleman lives in a one-story limestone house tucked between the olive trees Gates planted. Bougainvillea and plumbago flowers grace her patio. From an armchair in a spacious, light-filled living room, she greets me, wearing a black thobe with blue embroidery. "This is what I'm going to be buried in," she remarks good-humoredly.

Aileen Coleman (right) with Dr. Eleanor Soltau at the hospital's first location.

In 2024, on the occasion of his silver jubilee, Jordan's King Abdullah II honored Coleman with a silver medallion recognizing her more than fifty years of service in the Hashemite Kingdom. Even now, she continues to serve the Bedouin, visiting families in their tents twice a month though she is wheelchair-bound.

Coleman began her ministry in Sharjah, in the present-day United Arab Emirates. When she moved to Bethlehem to work at Baraka Hospital, she learned the importance of long-term disease care and fell in love with the Bedouin. She spent decades becoming as Bedouin as possible to reach the community with God's love, and has been a foster mother to at least nine Bedouin children.

The key to serving them physically and spiritually "is loving them, and not trying to change their Bedouin way of life," she says. "We're the ones who have got to change. It took me a long time to realize that."

Because of its openly Christian witness, Annoor has earned the local reputation of "the preaching hospital." A popular Bible-based film plays continuously in the clinic's waiting room. Five evenings a week, inpatients can choose to attend meetings where hymns are sung and scripture shared.

As one of Annoor's founders, Coleman has been embraced by all, in spite of religious differences. In the 1970s, during a civil war that pitted the Jordanian regime against the Palestinian Liberation Organization, a local tribe pledged protection to Coleman and Soltau and their hospital. When Coleman was in a near-fatal car accident in 1996, fifteen Bedouin men donated blood. The late King Hussein himself paid her hospital bill.

When I ask Coleman what brings patients, volunteers, and doctors from all over the world to Annoor, she answers simply. "Love," she says. "We love them."

WHILE WE'RE WALKING to and from Coleman's home, Heather Klassen, Herb's wife and Annoor's director of nursing, tells me about the changing face of TB in Jordan. When she came to Annoor in 1984, most of the inpatients were Bedouin. But current statistics from Jordan's Ministry of Health indicate that more than 50 percent of TB patients nationwide are Syrian, Bengali, or Filipino.

"We now have very few TB inpatients that are Bedouin, and for that reason, we have other outreaches," she says.

For twenty years, the Klassens staffed one of these outreaches, a clinic in Ras An-Naqab, 185 miles south of Mafraq. This location – which overlooks the vast sands of Wadi Rum – was opened in 1990 at the encouragement of Princess Shareefa Zein, a cousin of the late King Hussein who has supported Annoor's work among the Bedouin from the time she heard of it in the late 1980s.

Today the Naqab team serves twenty to forty patients every Friday in clinic. On other days, they visit Bedouin in remote areas, providing support for families with children who have disabilities and palliative care for those who are dying. They also run an income-generating workshop for local women, using sheep wool and camel hair to spin and weave using traditional methods.

"I want to show forgotten and desperate people that God really cares for them as a loving father," says the Dutch nurse who leads the Naqab outreach.

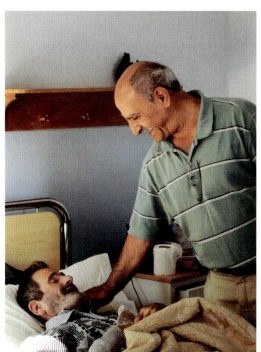

Abu Steve with a patient.

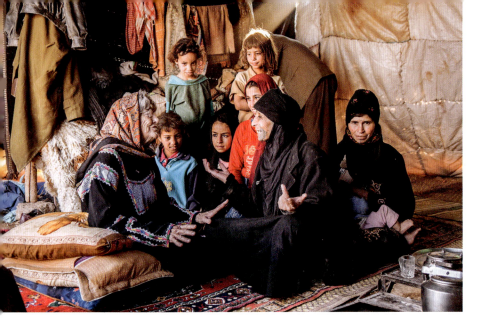

nurse; a Lebanese-British man; and three Jordanians. They read Jesus' words in Matthew 25:40: "Truly I tell you, whatever you did for one of the least of these brothers and sisters of mine, you did for me." After a brief prayer, the team loads into two vehicles and drives east.

The rising sun bleaches the highway to Zimla, one of several remote communities the dental team serves. After about thirty minutes the road turns to dirt. On either side, low shrubs grow between scattered chunks of basalt. A man herds his flock of sheep, backdropped by tents. Orchards appear on the horizon – olives, apricots, peaches, and persimmons – and then the dental truck, parked near a black and white striped tent.

From 1999 to 2019, Annoor operated a clinic in Ruwayshid, a town near the Jordan-Iraq border. Now, twice a month, a small team of hospital staff drives 125 miles from Mafraq to Ruwayshid to follow up with former patients. Along this route, they also visit families in their homes – whether tents or brick-and-mortar dwellings.

Her favorite part of her job, says the Norwegian nurse who leads this outreach, is the chance to visit children with disabilities in their homes, to encourage their mothers, to educate patients about breast cancer and diabetes, and to offer prayer.

"We want to see the people transformed," she says. "We want to see the dysfunctional families transformed. We want to see the drug addiction come to an end and the kids with disabilities treated right and included and not hidden away."

In 2013, Annoor acquired an unusual piece of equipment that enabled a third outreach: a twenty-five-foot mobile dental clinic, originally intended for use in North Korea but marooned in Dubai. Eventually, the truck was sent to Mafraq, where it serves inpatients and communities lacking local dental care.

On Saturday morning, I meet a diverse group of volunteers beneath the palm trees outside the clinic: two dentists, one Mexican and one Ecuadorian; a Syrian dental assistant; a Chinese

After greeting the queue, the team enters the truck to prepare for the day's work. The dentists can treat two patients at a time. A third can wait inside, giving volunteers the opportunity to interact and show God's love.

"God will do his work," one of them says.

Outside, two young women invite me into their family's tent. Sitting on rugs covering the dirt, we chat while drinking tiny glasses of sweet black tea and swatting flies away from a baby. I feel the infectious joy I've observed in Annoor's staff this weekend, the love that motivates their service among people often invisible to broader society.

As TB rates in Jordan have diminished since the 1960s, Coleman's dreams for the future are undimmed. She envisions households of Bedouin spreading the Good News in their own communities.

"I have seen some of this beginning," she says. "To God be the glory."

Aileen Coleman visits a Bedouin family in their home.

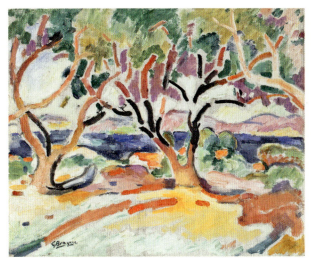

Georges Braque, *Olive Trees*, oil on canvas, 1907

The Stump
(Athens, Greece)

The mayor, I think, had it trucked in—this stump
Of an ancient olive tree. The muscled torso
In torsion like some wrestling Greek hero's
Statue found without its limbs—a lump
Of twisted xylem. For years I thought it dead—
Why had they planted a dead stump? The daisies
Sprang up around it in sunny waves. Taxis
Flowed on either side of the traffic island
It was marooned on like a shipwrecked mast.
And then, last spring, a crown of pale green shoots
Came arrowing out of it—I was flabbergasted,
It seemed a miracle! Now it's going gangbusters,
Branches in all directions. It's like the bed
The hero came home to, that he'd built himself,
And his wife had wept for years on like a life raft,
And the wonder wasn't that it was not moved—
(An inside joke)—but that it was still alive.

A. E. STALLINGS

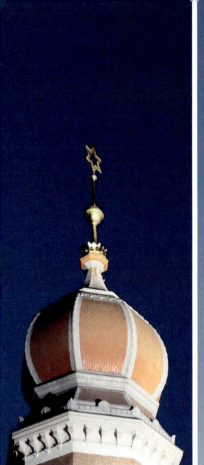 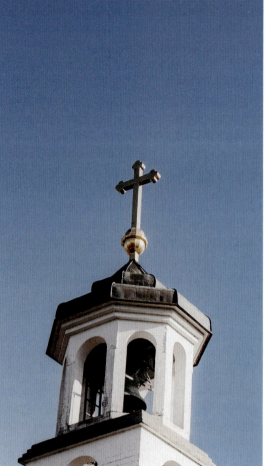 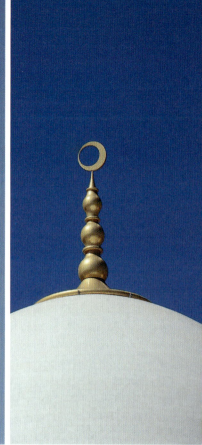

Abraham's Warring Children

After October 7, can a Muslim-Christian-Jewish center in Abu Dhabi make any difference?

KELSEY OSGOOD

"Are you still going to go?" I got this question a lot on October 8, 2023. It was Simchas Torah, the day Jews celebrate the conclusion of the yearly cycle of Torah reading, normally one of the most exuberant and joyful of our holidays. But that day, despite most of my neighbors in my Orthodox Jewish community in New York having their phones off in accordance with our religious observance, news of the massacre of civilians in southern Israel had been trickling in, and nobody was feeling particularly exuberant. In synagogue, parents sat with tense expressions and bloodshot eyes, attempting to hide their distress from the many young children present. One friend, father to a toddler and husband to a pregnant wife, wept as he danced

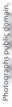

with the Torah: he was scheduled to fly out to meet his military reserve unit that evening, leaving his young and growing family behind.

So when I told people I had a flight that evening to Riyadh, Saudi Arabia – until fairly recently, a very unlikely destination for an American, let alone a Jewish American female solo traveler – their reactions ranged from skeptical to terrified. Mostly, I brushed off their concerns, though a tiny, doubtful part of me wondered if to go through with my plans wouldn't be very foolish indeed. I thought of the moment when, upon filling out my visa application, I'd come to a disclaimer about how it was a crime to bring materials offensive to Islam into the country, and I'd wondered briefly what would happen if I accidentally packed my daily prayerbook, with its reams of Hebrew text inside. Still, the trip – to meet a woman I'd been interviewing for my book on religious conversion, an American who'd relocated to Saudi Arabia in her early twenties – was years in the making. If I didn't go now, I figured, I never would.

There was also another reason to make the journey: I'd been assigned to write a story for a major newspaper about the Abrahamic Family House (AFH), a newly constructed center in Abu Dhabi where a church, a mosque, and a synagogue sat on a shared campus. The center also shared a coffee and gift shop and public areas with media projects like video installations on display. It ran programming events, too, some decidedly theological in nature (like lectures on the Prophet Muhammad) while others, such as weaving baskets or learning sign language, confusingly related to faith only tangentially. I'd first read about the center in 2020, and had kept tabs on the project for years, hoping to cover it somehow. When I saw the chance to make a stop in Abu Dhabi, I scrambled to pitch the piece, and was thrilled when it was accepted.

As I'd researched the Abrahamic Family House before my departure, I'd become very familiar with its many critics and their complaints. The most common objection was that it was simple "faith-washing": like golf in Saudi Arabia, the AFH served as a shiny symbol of tolerance designed to deflect attention from the human rights abuses in the region. People in this camp generally pointed out that the center, like many "public" institutions in the United Arab Emirates, was owned and funded by the government, and therefore must have been built on the backs of underpaid and overworked foreign laborers, a longstanding issue in the region (one which, in fairness, the government has tried to address in recent years).

There were also questions of how well the individual institutions at the AFH could fulfill their sacred obligations, given that the official religion of the nation is Islam. Could a Catholic church there effectively evangelize, for example? But also, seeing as how the UAE government – authoritarian by nature, and made up almost exclusively of wealthy sheikhs – carefully monitored and restricted speech by imams under the guise of preventing extremism, how could even the Muslim cleric freely minister? The situation for local Jews, meanwhile, was a whole other ball of wax. When I'd mentioned the center to my husband, he looked at me sideways. "How many Jews even *live* there?" he'd asked. (Answer: though the growth of the community has been much ballyhooed since the signing of the Abraham Accords, estimates hover around a meager one thousand, a majority of whom live in Dubai, which means actually worshipping regularly at the AFH would be challenging.)

Kelsey Osgood is a writer whose work has appeared in The New Yorker, Time, *and* Harper's Magazine. *She has written two books,* How to Disappear Completely *(Overlook, 2013), and* Godstruck *(Penguin Random House, 2025).*

The other major strain of criticism was largely theological: namely, that this interfaith project – and indeed, by extension, *any* interfaith project – was untenable, if not immoral, because from the point of view of the one Objective Truth (whatever the critic understood that to be), any attempt to play nice with people who didn't recognize Objective Truth was tantamount to religious suicide. This viewpoint was voiced, briefly and indelicately, by the occasional Muslim commenter on the site's Instagram page ("Religion is with Allah, Islam," one such comment read, "and you will not get what you want no matter what you do"). It was also stated, less briefly but still stridently, by Eric Sammons, the editor-in-chief of the traditionalist Catholic magazine *Crisis*, who filmed a thirty-minute video in which he called the AFH "another sign that interreligious dialogue has transformed into religious indifference." (He also sniped at the center's aesthetic: it "looks almost like the Fortress of Solitude from Superman," he said.)

The first round of criticisms I found relatively easy to ignore. Though of course I would never scoff at human rights abuses, it seemed to me that, unlike golf in Saudi Arabia, building centers for religious tolerance *was* actually addressing the historical charge that the UAE wasn't a welcoming place for non-Muslims. (The country did this in other ways too: in 2024, a massive Hindu temple, unconnected to the Abrahamic Family House, opened outside Abu Dhabi, to serve the many Indian nationals who live and work there.)

But the theological dissent was a little harder to dismiss. Like any neurotic author worth her salt, I spent an inordinate amount of time imagining the various reasons people would hate my book. My biggest point of self-consciousness was that I'd be charged with promoting what's called "moralistic therapeutic deism," a term that describes viewing spirituality as primarily about making people feel nice and be baseline ethical, rather than about living in accordance with the occasionally demanding challenges of a specific belief.

Perhaps it was my biggest fear because it was kind of true: I *did* actually believe that having faith is conducive to wellbeing, even if I also believed, paradoxically, that some of that wellbeing comes out of the experience of sublimating the self and its desires, and I do think it's probably more important that people have faith at all than that they have the *right* faith. But I'm also an Orthodox Jew, which means I adhere to a strict set of rules that I believe are divinely mandated, nonnegotiable, and specific (mostly) to Jews. Can these two ideas coexist in a person? Does recognizing the sociological benefits of religion undermine one's understanding of it as objective, sacred truth? And further, is it unforgivable heresy to support or even advocate for religious diversity – as different faiths can reap these benefits in different ways – as a believer in the

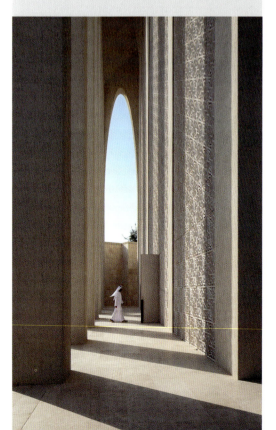

The Abrahamic Family House in Abu Dhabi was designed by Ghanaian-British architect Sir David Frank Adjaye. The symbolic designs of the three buildings, which are constructed from local limestone, celebrate each of the three Abrahamic faiths.

The Imam Al-Tayeb Mosque faces Mecca and features *mashrabiya*, or traditional Islamic latticework, which lets in light while keeping the structure ventilated.

supremacy of one's own truth? Or is appreciating that diversity the more realistic, the kinder, even the more theologically accurate thing to do?

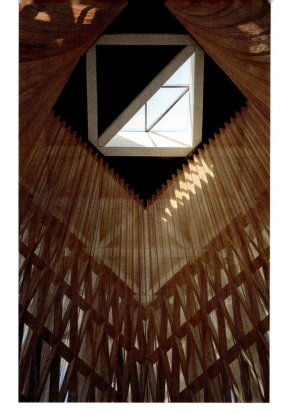

I USED TO THINK that Judaism is uniquely hospitable to pluralism. For all the charges of exclusivity leveled at my chosen faith, it doesn't insist that one must be Jewish to be righteous on earth or saved in death. In one of my favorite passages of the Tosefta, the rabbis argue over whether non-Jews are also granted a share in what we call *olam haba*, or the world to come. Citing a mention of the nations who "forget" God in the psalms, Rabbi Eliezer says that they are not, but Rabbi Yehoshua disagrees: "If the text had said 'the wicked shall return to *sheol*' . . . and [then] was quiet, then I would say like you said," he retorts. "But now the verse said those who forget God. Behold, there are saints among the nations [and] they have a share in the world to come." Figures ranging from the medieval Sephardic poet and physician Yehudah Halevi to the seventeenth-century Talmudist Yaakov Emden even wrote admiringly of Christianity and Islam as forces for good. "Whereas the nations before them worshipped idols, denied God's existence, and thus did not recognize God's power or retribution," Rabbi Emden wrote, "the rise of Christianity and Islam served to spread among the nations, to the furthest ends of the earth, the knowledge that there is one God who rules the world, who rewards and punishes and reveals himself to man."

Closer to our current era, the late, beloved Rabbi Lord Jonathan Sacks asked hopefully in his 2002 book *The Dignity of Difference*, "Does our sense of the all-encompassing nature of the divine lead us to recognize the integrity of the search for God by those outside our faith?" He unequivocally believed it should, but his argument was a little *too* open for some: for the second edition in 2003, he amended his previous suggestion that God had "spoken" to different groups of people via different faiths, a statement that saw him summoned before a consortium of displeased Orthodox rabbis.

Through my personal and professional interfaith interactions – professionally because I often cover other faiths in my writing; personal because I like to have friends with different beliefs – I've come to question this assumption of pluralistic superiority, though. In the Torah, the ideal Gentile is Noah; he is the namesake for the so-called seven Noahide laws, which form the basis for non-Jewish ethical behavior. Per Rabbi Emden, many Christians and Muslims get there anyway, despite what Jews would consider their extra-textual beliefs, but for some rabbis, a more ideal scenario would be for them to actually identify and worship as Noahides and discard any post-Torah ideas of prophecy, which would more or less relegate them to cosmic supporting characters. Thus it should come as no surprise that a sizable number of the few self-identifying Noahides out there end up converting (many to Judaism, but some to Christianity). To frame it differently, if I'm allowing Christians entrance into theoretical heaven, but not validating their belief in Christ, perhaps that's just as offensive as the reverse, in

The skylight of the Moses Ben Maimon Synagogue mimics a chuppah, a canopy used in Jewish wedding ceremonies, while the crisscross architectural motif represents the palm trees used to build a sukkah, a temporary shelter used during the Jewish festival of Sukkot.

which a Christian says yes, God made a covenant with Jews, but you won't be spared in the afterlife. My own needle, it turns out, seems to be just as hard to thread as, say, the one my close Catholic friend, a devout consecrated virgin, wields when she lays out the church's official stance that God's bond with the Jews should be respected, "but of course we hope everyone will ultimately become Catholic." It is as hard, too, as the needle Muslims must thread when trying to internalize the Koranic idea that there should be no coercion in religion alongside the idea of Islam as the one true faith. Logically, isn't it somehow ungenerous to believe one holds the only truth and *not* try to convince others to see it too?

Besides, there are limits to my own pluralism. Interfaith initiatives are well and good, but they can also be uniquely simplistic and, well, corny (see again: the basket weavers of Abu Dhabi). A few years ago, I sat in on an interfaith discussion between Latter-day Saints and Catholics, listening to the participants marvel excitedly over the similarities between the two faiths, even though it seemed to me that an equal if not greater number of similarities could be enumerated between *any* two faiths. Plus, as Rabbi Sacks wrote, focusing so much on the things we have in common might lead us to neglect the things that we *don't* share, which could mean that we're underprepared to address those differences when they inevitably arise. Must we emphasize our commonalities in order to coexist, or can we see our points of departure, awkward though discussion of them might be, as *enhancing* the world and our relationships?

There's also a bright line where my kumbaya self ends and my Objective Truth one begins, and that's when it comes to anything Jewish. Though the Jewish canon is vast and its number of opinions legion, it's pretty well accepted in the Orthodox world that all Jews should at the very least keep Shabbat, the laws of kosher, and those of ritual purity, which govern sexual relations (there are myriad *cultural* points of diversion, but that's a different conversation). Once, a close friend from college, who is nonobservant but who has a strong Jewish identity, stopped by my house on a Saturday afternoon. My oldest son asked her, in the blunt manner of young children, if she was Jewish. She said yes.

"Then why are you driving on Shabbat?" he asked.

"Well, we're what's called Reform Jews," she told him. "Your mom has probably told you about how some Jews do some things differently!" She continued on in this vein for a while, before wrapping up with some broad-strokes inter-Jewish platitudes. But this friend would perhaps be surprised – and maybe even offended – to know that I would *never* tell my children that it's okay for Jews to not keep Shabbat, regardless of their denominational affiliation.

The project of being a religious person who's respectful of, or even one who *loves*, the world's vast cornucopia of belief is complicated. But it's one I'll admit I've always enjoyed. To dig deep into my own tradition's texts, to watch my companions of other faiths wrestle with their own religions' views: it feels like a logic puzzle, a stretching and strengthening of mental muscles, that ideally leaves us all better off in the end. Sure, it can be messy, but is anything worthwhile not? And yet, as the year after that fateful Simchas Torah would teach me, it could always be messier.

MY BOOK SUBJECT picked me up at the airport in Riyadh when I arrived; in the car, while driving me to the hotel, she said she'd wondered if I'd had second thoughts about coming, given what had happened in Israel.

"It did make me nervous," I said.

"You can tell anyone you're Jewish here," she said. She was working for an international organization that was about to host a major investment conference in the city the week after I departed, with many Jews from all over the world in attendance. "Literally *no one* cares."

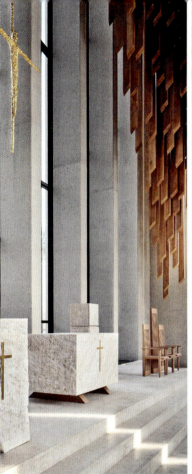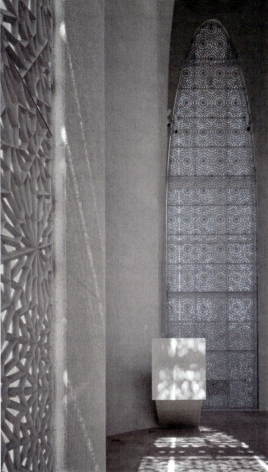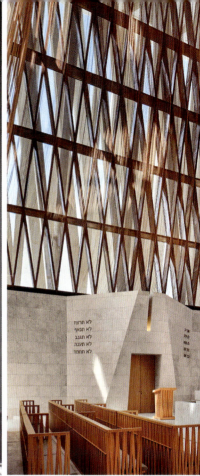

Outside of the constant CNN coverage of the impending, seemingly inevitable conflict on the TV in my hotel's lobby, I saw nothing in Riyadh that made me feel like I was in a region on the brink: no protests, no marches, no Palestinian flags flown in solidarity. No one mentioned it to me, but then again, I didn't follow the suggestion that I tell people I was Jewish, so maybe they were leaving things unsaid, too. During the daytime, a tour guide drove me into the desert to ride camels, pointing out where the world's biggest Six Flags was set to be built on the way; at night, in my hotel room, I'd watch endless clips of people expressing support for Jews – elderly Japanese people singing "Oseh Shalom" in Tokyo, say, or gay American comedians giving sassy monologues denouncing Hamas – in hopes of feeling less isolated.

My flight to Abu Dhabi was at a punishing hour of the morning, so I arrived at the Abrahamic Family House sweaty and exhausted when it opened. It was a Friday, two days before Israel began its ground offensive in Gaza; locals who usually hosted Shabbat meals in the area had canceled their services as a precaution. A person previously affiliated with the AFH had told me not to worry: the center was filled with security "both seen and unseen," which had the curious effect of making me feel somewhat less safe than I had before.

In the lobby, I was met by a trio of female handlers, two who worked for the AFH and one public-relations representative, whose distant demeanor reminded me of something I'd read about the space: "Atop the one-story volume sits the central plaza," wrote Izzy Kornblatt in *Architectural Record*, which "is far too hot under the brutal equatorial sun to allow for lingering during daylight hours. Actually, it isn't just the plaza. One does not feel welcome to linger anywhere in the Abrahamic House, except,

The Church of Saint Francis (left), which faces east, features hundreds of vertical hanging slats that frame the chancel. Also shown are details from the mosque (center) and the synagogue (right).

perhaps, the welcome center's exhibitions."

To a degree, I could see his point. As we wandered throughout the complex, I clocked the ways the design managed to be sumptuous but also more than a little austere. The abstract crucifix in the church, named for Saint Francis of Assisi, was made in Milan of twenty-four karat gold. The carpet in Eminence Ahmed El-Tayeb Mosque was plush on my bare feet – shoes weren't allowed inside, in deference to Muslim practice – and the place was pristine; its latticework façade, done in the delicate style of North African *mashrabiya,* cast dappled shadows on the floor that looked unmistakably like snowflakes. There was even a touch of ridiculous luxury: each house of worship, the tour guide told me, has its own signature scent diffused throughout the space.

But I disagreed with Kornblatt's later comment that the facility prioritized the tourist over the worshiper. Each of the spaces was fully functioning from a religious perspective: you could pray five times a day in the mosque, *lein* from a Torah scroll in the synagogue, and baptize a baby at the church. (Indeed, the AFH even had its own mikvah, which actually might make the area a more livable place for Orthodox Jews than some locales.) That a majority of the people who came to pray there were Muslims rather than Jews and Christians seemed to me not damnable but just a matter of demographics.

We wound our way back through the front exhibition area, where videos of people praying in different languages played on loop (they looked staged, but the tour guide told me they were documentary-style). An elderly Australian man, who told us he was Orthodox Christian, kept trying to chat us up every time we bumped into him. "We're all going to the same place," he pontificated, "we just use different maps," a line so extraordinarily on-the-nose I would have assumed he'd been paid to say it, had my guides not kept trying to rebuff his overtures. As a person prone to cynicism, I kept wondering how it was that, despite all the flaws of this place, I found myself inexplicably welling up with tears. When the guides and PR rep departed, I slunk back into the synagogue, which was empty save for a single security guard, grabbed a crisp new prayerbook from the shelf, sat on the sleek oak bench, and wept.

IN THE YEAR and a half since my visit to the Abrahamic Family House, its pluralistic dream has seemed farther away than ever. Jews have been torn apart waiting for news of their hostages; Gaza, meanwhile, lies in ruins. Talk of coexistence between Israel and Palestine, even from many who'd previously championed a two-state solution, has become a whisper. Meanwhile, a rabbi ministering to the community in Dubai, Zvi Kogan, was abducted and murdered in November 2024, more than a year after my visit. To its credit, the government swiftly captured the perpetrators, but the vision of the country as a safe haven for Jews, or maybe anyone else different, had been blemished.

As for the piece: the editor sat on it for months. She finally admitted she was waffling. It just felt too weird to talk about an interfaith center in the Middle East without giving greater attention to the increasing conflagration between Jews and Muslims, she suggested. Eventually, she decided to kill the piece.

I understood why. How could we pretend that things were fine even in that tiny plot of earth, let alone in the region where it stands, or maybe even the world? How silly, how delusional, to believe there could be anywhere we could all get along. How ridiculous and starry-eyed to try to downplay our hatreds, ignore our grievances, extinguish our rage.

But I'll tell you this: I've sometimes thought since my return home that, uncomfortable though it was, there was nowhere I'd rather have been than sitting on that bench in that imperfect, empty monument to togetherness, crying and praying for something new.

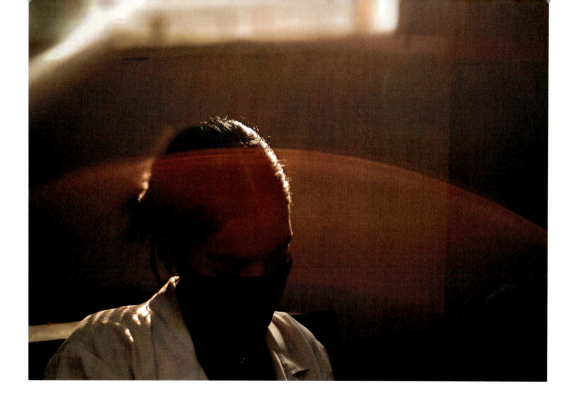

Who Cares for the Carers?

Hidden in plain sight, foriegn health aides in UK nursing homes face exploitation.

HAZEL THOMPSON

IN 2019, when she was twenty-five, Farah (not her real name) moved to the United Kingdom to pursue a master's degree in business. Despite already holding bachelor's and master's degrees in engineering and technology from universities in India, she faced significant challenges in finding stable employment. The expiration of her student visa meant that she would need to secure a work visa in order to remain in the country with her husband (whose right to remain depended on hers) and their new baby.

Farah submitted more than three hundred work applications before finally receiving a job offer from a care home in Greater Manchester in December 2022. This offer came via Indeed, a reputable recruiting website. The care home company assured her of a certificate of sponsorship, a crucial document linking her immigration status to her employer. The UK government grants these work visas through employer sponsorship, a program that allows foreign nationals to work in the United Kingdom for employers that have a

Hazel Thompson is a British photojournalist and filmmaker who has worked for the Guardian *and* New York Times *as well as various NGOs, primarily focusing on trafficking, slavery, and sexual violence.*

government-approved sponsor license. This means that if someone's employment is terminated, he or she can lose the right to remain.

"During the interview, I made it clear I couldn't work six days straight because of our baby," Farah explains. "They assured me that we could manage with a combination of shifts shared with my husband, telling me I can work four days and he can work two days, and we would get one day together off at home."

Although entry-level care work was far afield from what Farah had studied for, she was glad of the opportunity, and her initial experiences working in care were good. "I received good training and support," she says, and the management was pleasant and accommodating.

However, as time passed, the promise faded. The job made escalating demands on her time and Farah and her husband found themselves shuffled into grueling shift rotations and schedules that stripped them of any family time. Farah expressed her concerns to management but was met with indifference or hostility. When the couple tried to refuse shifts, their hours became, if anything, even more punishing.

Under UK law, a care worker who is sponsored must work a minimum of 37.5 hours per week and be paid a minimum of £11.44 per hour. The worker must have at least eleven hours of rest between working days and at least one full day off each week, or two full days every two weeks, with at least 5.6 weeks' paid holiday per year. These regulations bore no relationship to the schedule Farah and her husband were required to perform.

In the midst of this turmoil, sickness arrived. An outbreak of vomiting and diarrhea swept through the care home, leaving Farah, her husband, and their baby daughter very ill. Even so, the management's primary concern was to force employees back to work, threatening their jobs if they refused (and apparently without regard for the patients they might expose).

Later, Covid-19 struck the care home, affecting patients and staff. Farah and her husband tested positive but their illnesses were quickly dismissed, and despite their being very unwell, the management demanded they return to duty. "That's when our real struggle happened," Farah says. She recalls her manager throwing the phone, shouting, "I have given you a free visa and I didn't know you have a baby, why have you not left your baby with your family in India?" She says he threatened to fabricate a story about her that would put her directly in jail. "He got very aggressive. He was shouting and I was shivering through the phone."

At this point Farah's husband resigned. But Farah did not, as the whole family's right to reside and work in the United Kingdom was dependent on her visa. The work environment continued to sour.

"Sometimes they made me work nine days in a row with back-to-back shifts. After five months, I had not had a day off and no weekends," Farah says. Meanwhile, she was shouted at and humiliated in front of the other staff.

At the end of these five months, Farah requested to take two weeks of her annual leave, so she could visit her family in India for the first time in four years and so her family could meet her now two-year-old child for the first time. Her child also required some specialist eye surgery back in India. At first management refused, but then reluctantly granted her ten days.

ON THE FAMILY'S RETURN to the United Kingdom, Farah faced a new challenge; the care home refused to give her any shifts. "For two weeks I called them and I asked them why you are not putting me on the rota, as they were stopping any income, and they said it's punishment because I took annual leave."

Farah and her husband's financial situation became so difficult that they were unable to pay rent or bills. They borrowed money from her parents back in India (who did not have much themselves) to make ends meet, and were soon at risk of homelessness.

In December 2023, a British colleague working at the care home, perhaps more aware of national law and resources, pointed Farah in the direction of the Gangmasters and Labour Abuse Authority (GLAA), a UK government agency focused on preventing and tackling labor exploitation. She also got in touch with a charity called Justice and Care, which partners with police forces in the United Kingdom to support the victims of egregious labor violations. I have reported alongside Justice and Care on a number of stories over the last seven years, including being present on police investigations. In the last two years the organization has seen a surge of exploitation cases within the care sector.

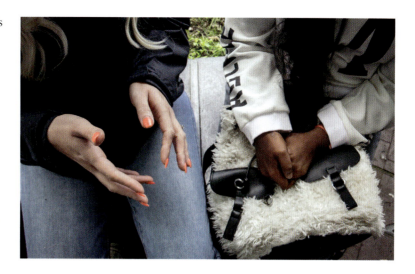

Justice and Care connected Farah with one of its "victim navigators," Melissa (also a pseudonym, due to the nature of her work), who taught Farah about her rights and how to report her employer's exploitation. Melissa guided Farah through the process of formally reporting her treatment to the GLAA, which started to investigate the care home.

Other care workers at the home made anonymous complaints, but when UK Visa Immigration (UKVI) and GLAA came to interview the staff individually they did not want to talk, possibly due to fear of repercussions. When a company has its UKVI sponsorship license revoked, it cannot continue to employ international workers, leaving those workers only sixty days to either find new sponsorship or leave the country – an outcome similar to the threat their employers might use against them.

After Farah's employer found out she was the whistleblower, the company tried to force her to sign a legal statement to retract her complaint, threatening her that all the other staff would lose their jobs and livelihoods because of her. The management refused to give a reference for any future employment or sponsorship.

The investigation came to a close with little remuneration for Farah. The care home did have its sponsorship license suspended for a short time. However, after an investigation by the UKVI the company made some changes and was given its sponsorship license back. Farah, who has stayed in touch with some old colleagues, does take comfort in knowing that at least working conditions have improved for them somewhat after this intervention.

Sadly, Farah's story is not unique. In my thirty-year career as a photojournalist and filmmaker, I have traveled to nearly seventy countries to gather stories. My calling is to investigate, document, and expose the disturbing truths around modern slavery, human trafficking, and exploitation. And yet, even I was shocked to learn of the exploitation happening right on my own doorstep here in the United Kingdom.

There is a huge demand for people willing to

Melissa guides Farah through the process of reporting her employer's exploitative treatment.

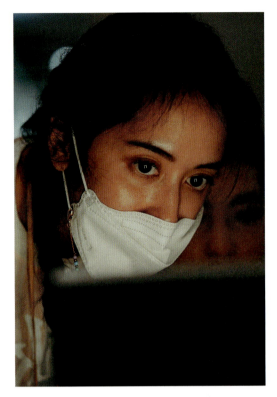

work in care, a vocation that many native Brits find unattractive. This has been amplified since Brexit, as there has been a significant drop in the movement of European Union nationals coming to work in the sector. The latest government figures show almost 106,000 visas were granted to care workers in 2023, a number that has tripled from the same period in 2022. People from India, Nigeria, Zimbabwe, Ghana, Bangladesh, and Pakistan topped the list of nationalities traveling to the United Kingdom to plug the labor gap. Although there are some safeguards in place, many of those coming to work in the care sector have a poor understanding of their rights.

On top of that, many of these workers are misled as to the true costs of their visa. A common situation, says Melissa, is that a supposed middleman "will charge illegal fees for the visa. This could be anything from £10,000 to £50,000 for a visa that actually costs just over £300." To pay these illegitimate costs, many international workers sell family assets such as land or businesses in their home countries.

Nine out of ten cases that come through the GLAA are from the care sector, Melissa says. Victims "confide in us about the struggle to find alternative sponsorships, all while carrying the burden of feeding their families. They fear letting their families down back home, to tell them it hasn't worked out; it's very embarrassing and shameful for them."

Melissa emphasizes the psychological as well as financial toll such exploitation takes, recounting a stark example:

> We had a woman who came to the United Kingdom with her husband and two children and paid £28,000 for her sponsored job, using her dad's pension money to pay the illegal fee. When she complained about her hours, she was told, "You're here on my visa; you'll do as you're told." The woman received a lot of psychological abuse as well, and one day her husband came home to find her writing a suicide note. Luckily, he managed to stop her.

J USTICE AND CARE considers these kinds of employment pressures so acute as to call them "slavery." According to the GLAA, forced and compulsory labor is defined as "all work or service which is exacted from any person under the threat of a penalty and for which the person has not offered themselves voluntarily." The agency's latest report focuses solely on labor exploitation, excluding other forms of modern slavery, such as sexual exploitation and forced begging.

One of the most striking findings from the report is its insights into what factors make victims of exploitation most vulnerable. The most common vulnerability stems from immigration status being linked to employment. Fear of deportation or job loss keeps many silent even in the face of unacceptable working conditions.

As Melissa notes, "Many of these international workers believe that their sponsors hold the power to deport them. This fear keeps them in a place of compliance, even when exploitation is at play."

The care sector has emerged as a critical area of concern in the GLAA's report, consistently marked as the most reported sector for modern slavery indicators. In the most recent quarter alone, care home and social care settings accounted for 47 percent of all reports and referrals related to forced labor.

The report highlights a range of exploitation types, with pay issues featuring prominently. This includes inadequate or withheld wages and unexplained deductions. The next most common form of exploitation reported was being made to work long hours, a condition often linked to jobs in the care sector that require workers to travel between various locations during shifts.

Another critical finding suggests a direct correlation between the provision of accommodation and exploitation. In 33 percent of cases, victims were forced to live in substandard conditions controlled by their employers. This factor creates an additional layer of vulnerability, leaving these workers fearful of being evicted.

Most reported victims were female. Conversely, the exploiters were predominantly male, and mainly of British nationality. This points to a troubling power dynamic as well.

I SPOKE TO ANDREW BROWN, the National Investigations Lead at the GLAA, whose role involves tracking the rise of labor exploitation and modern slavery in the UK care sector. His insights shed light on the systemic issues that allow these violations to persist.

The GLAA has successfully implemented a licensing scheme in sectors like horticulture, agriculture, food processing, and shell fishing, focusing on stringent oversight through rigorous inspection processes. However, in the adult care sector there is a troubling gap in regulatory measures from the government, as it is not one of GLAA's regulated sectors. The increasing demand for care services, coupled with low interest in that work from British citizens and generally undesirable pay and conditions, "creates a perfect storm for exploitation," he states.

The sharp rise in exploitation cases follows the government's decision in February 2020 to make foreign social care workers eligible for temporary visas that were previously reserved for higher-paid workers. In the following eighteen months, 180,000 health and care visas were granted, a rate almost three times higher than before, filling more than 165,000 vacancies.

Between August 2020, when the health and care worker visa was launched, and March 2024, the latest month covered in the report, the number of care providers with visa sponsorship licenses ballooned from just over 250 to more than 3,200. Since then, nearly 200 have been removed from the Home Office register for bad practice.

Brown notes that the partnership between the GLAA and organizations like Justice and Care has proven invaluable in providing a support network for victims of exploitation. He hopes to achieve better industry regulation and more collaboration among agencies. "We need to drive toward regulations that safeguard workers – both from predatory recruitment practices and from the cycle of exploitation fostered by the current sponsorship system," he says. He also hopes to raise awareness among prospective workers for their own protection.

Melissa also hopes to raise awareness among the people who rely on these care workers, often hidden in plain sight. "When you visit care homes or meet care workers, check in with them. Are they well? Are they overworked?"

With Melissa's help, Farah found a new sponsor and began to rebuild her life. Both she and her husband work for a different company now, and their daughter is thriving.

COMMUNITY SNAPSHOT

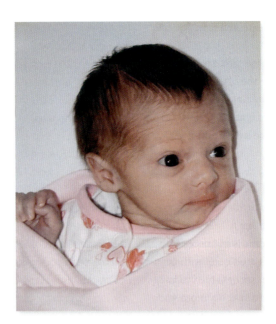

Little Person, Big Welcome

Bringing home a baby on the Bruderhof is no small affair.

MAUREEN SWINGER

We stood in the doorway, gawking. Our apartment was almost unrecognizable. We had hurried out the door in the wee hours of Tuesday, a family of two, and now we were back on Thursday, returning at a slower pace – in fact, fairly gliding along so as not to jiggle the very tiny third family member sound asleep in her car seat. Every surface was covered in flowers, cards, and gifts: a welcome sign draped down the wall, courtesy of the kindergarten class, pink balloons on the ceiling, adorable baby clothes hung across the curtain rods, and the counter laden with a heaping It's-a-Girl basket with a pink champagne bottle peeking out the top.

I was amazed, but not surprised. This was our first time on the receiving end of such largesse, but I can't count how many times I had the fun of preparation, scurrying around while the family was at the hospital, deep cleaning, bringing practical supplies for mom and baby, arranging gifts, stocking the fridge, putting up decorations, and generally making the house into one giant welcome for a new arrival. It doesn't matter if it's a first child or a fifth. Any baby born on a Bruderhof community gets this reception – not just in tangible gifts, but in the love of a two-hundred-member family.

As I was reading the thirtieth congratulation card blurrily at two a.m. (being up anyway), I was filled with wordless gratitude, not only for our baby, but for the love surrounding her. When life is humming along, it's easy to forget about the strong network that undergirds a life of shared

Maureen and Jason's first daughter, 2008.

work and goods and time. But it rises up to support you all the same.

As useful as all the material gifts are, support comes in many forms, and one of its most beautiful forms is the "grandma," an older woman whose task it is to look after a new mom. If there's a biological grandmother anywhere within travel range, that's her prerogative. (This is in addition to the routine check-ins by medical professionals who are attuned to conditions like postpartum depression, and also happy to answer questions about nursing or sleep patterns.)

Being a new baby's grandma is not necessarily a hovering job; some moms need quiet with an occasional hello, and others are delighted to have company. I was in the latter camp; my mom was waiting in our house when we arrived home, folding back the crib blankets so her granddaughter could (hopefully) continue sleeping.

I love my mom every day of the week, but those days were truly next-level as we got to know our little person together, singing to her, cuddling her, helping her clear the five-pound mark. It started my mom down memory lane. As I was her first child and only daughter, who also began life as a bit of a lightweight, I heard all the fond comparisons.

To feed the baby, you must feed the mom; thus, here comes the dad at noon, toting an enormous tray of food – some healthy, some just plain good – made with great intentionality by one of the women in the communal kitchen. It's her task to cook for the people who require special diets, and then to provide daily lunches and dinners for new parents. The size of one raspberry cream cheese pie alone seemed to operate on the assumption that our household included ten people, not counting the one with no teeth.

It does present the chance to invite friends over to dote on the baby and help attack the pie. It's also a chance to share the joy of the newborn days with someone who might not often have the chance to hold a child.

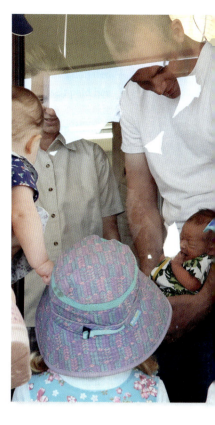

In a community the size of ours, two hundred individual visitors would be a little overwhelming. But everyone's keen to meet the kid, and one way we do that is to take the baby to a ground-floor room with a big window, and have the entire community stroll past to offer their congratulations in one go. There's a whole canon of lovely lullabies in the Bruderhof song repertoire, and often they will be sung by the people waiting their turn in the line. The window gets smudges from small noses pressing against the glass, and the baby's parents get aching cheeks from smiling proudly for so long.

My husband stood tall, cradling his little lady – from top to toe, she was as long as his forearm. If one more person had exclaimed, "Look at those eyes!" the buttons on his shirt would have popped off in all directions.

O UR BABY'S FIRST WEEKS went so well that I figured I would manage just fine next time around. The second baby had other plans. His colic had us taking shifts to pace around the house like trapped cats. We tried all recommended remedies to no avail. It got to the point where whenever he cried, I cried, and he cried more than he did anything else.

Maureen Swinger is an editor at Plough *and lives at the Fox Hill Bruderhof in Walden, New York, with her husband, Jason, and their three children.*

A family at the Danthonia Bruderhof introduces their new baby to the community.

My wonderful neighbor Becky stopped by and offered to take him for a spell one afternoon, but I was still in my managing-mom phase and turned her down politely. By the next morning, I ran across the lawn to her cottage, babe in arms. When she opened the door, I thrust him at her unceremoniously. She took him with a delighted grin, plopped him over her arm like a football, and the noise stopped instantly. Turns out she once had a son with colic, and it had lasted six months. I doubted my sanity would last six weeks.

Even today, when that former baby looks down on her from a great height, she still likes to kid me that he is really her baby whom she has just let me borrow for a bit. Interactions like these, lighthearted but genuine, help a child grow up in the confidence of wide-ranging kinship, like Wendell Berry's "membership" that extends beyond family ties.

There's one ceremony that parents look forward to especially – a more solemn welcome not just to a community, but to a church.

Of course, there's a biblical precedent for this; the second chapter of Luke describes Mary and Joseph taking eight-day-old Jesus to the temple "to present him to the Lord," and the accompanying prophecies and praise of Simeon and Anna as soon as they behold the baby.

Presentation of infants to the church is also an old Anabaptist tradition first mentioned in a letter from theologian Balthasar Hubmaier in 1525: "I like to assemble the congregation in the place of baptism, bringing the child. . . . As soon as his name has been given to him, the whole congregation on bended knee prays for the child, entrusting him to the hands of Christ, that he may be ever closer to the child and pray on his behalf."

This presentation reflects a deep theological point: Anabaptists believe that babies are born innocent, an untainted soul entering a tarnished world. Bruderhof founder Eberhard Arnold once wrote that "every child is a thought of God," and thus should be welcomed with reverence for the mystery of God's specific thought for that specific child.

A church blessing befits a baby whose family is also part of a wider church family. The parents will bring their child to the center of our meeting circle and put him in the arms of a pastor, who then speaks out a blessing and a prayer requesting God's guidance in the child's life. Sometimes the baby gets passed along to the grandparents, who add their own wishes for the child to grow in health, love, an understanding of God's path for him or her, and service to others. This is followed by a prayer in which all members take silent part, vowing to uphold the child and support his parents in the years ahead.

Our good friend and pastor Richard Scott gave the blessing for our son. He had baptized me, married us, and seen us through quite a few ups and downs already, so we were glad he was the one holding our baby, looking down at him as he spoke: "Now when we think of this little child, it reminds us how Jesus took the little children in his arms to receive them. He let them come to him, saying, 'Whoever receives this child in my name, receives me.' When anyone believes in Jesus, they are called children of God, and children of his Spirit."

We were happy with our son and daughter, born sixteen months apart but now as inseparable as twins. Number three arrived five years after we had packed the baby clothes away. Hearing again the prayer and promise, I felt a new, stronger sense of the big circle of faith surrounding us, into which God gave us this beautiful baby who will grow up with all the usual struggles and joys of childhood and adolescence. But we won't be going it alone, either in the struggle or the joy.

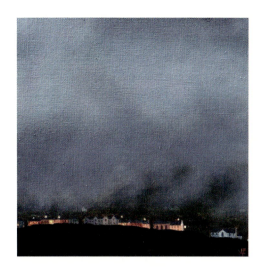

It Could Be Worse

It could be worse, my dear, it could be worse.
The world is ending—this was always true.
But that could be a blessing, not a curse.

We've made a sow's ear out of a silk purse,
The permafrost is neither, sea's less blue.
It could be worse, my dear, it could be worse.

In tragedy, the chorus moans in verse;
Prose is available to me and you,
And that could be a blessing, not a curse.

Some roles we improvise, and some rehearse;
Let's swell a progress, start a scene or two!
It could be worse, my dear, it could be worse:

Grudges, infants, fears, small things we nurse.
The future is a dream that will come true.
But that could be a blessing, not a curse.

Only by spending, will love reimburse—
The world is ending. But that's nothing new.
It could be worse, my dear, it could be worse,
And this could be a blessing, not a curse.

A. E. STALLINGS

Tim Goulding, *Evening Allihies Village 4*, acrylic and oil on canvas.

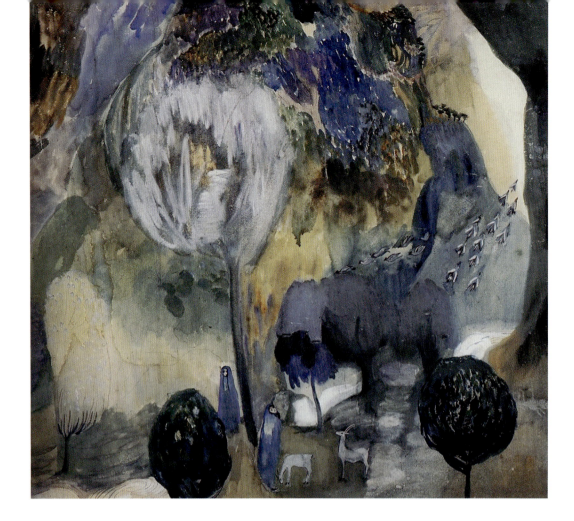

Armenia's Day of the Dead

These two short stories from Plough's *new book* To Go On Living *are set in an Armenian mountain village during the recent conflict there.*

NARINE ABGARYAN

Merelots

Ginamants Metaksia leaves her house bright and early, at the crack of dawn. A flock of village swallows, having abandoned their perches in the cypress trees, are swooping overhead, making notches on the canvas of the quickly brightening sky with their sharp-tipped wings. The first dew – dense, life-giving – falls, dispatching the night. A cricket, confused about the hour of the day, breaks into its drawling song: chirr-up, chirr-up, chirr-up.

"Good morning to you too, you poor soul," Metaksia greets him in her mind. The cricket, as if hearing her thoughts, cuts off and falls silent.

Today is Merelots, the day of the dead. Traditionally, people attend the memorial service first and only after that visit the graves of their

Martiros Sarian, *Blossoming Mountains*, 1905.

departed loved ones. There was a time when Metaksia also followed this tradition, but then she decided that it was not right to delay the visit to the dead – after all, what use do the departed have for liturgy when they have gone to a place where nothing worldly matters? Therefore, she figured, the proper way to go about it was to start the day of remembrance with a trip to the graveyard before attending to any other business. So as to completely dispel any doubts, she consulted the priest. He heard her out and nodded in agreement: "You do what you think is right; if you feel more at peace doing things in this order, then you should." Metaksia certainly felt more at peace doing things in this order.

The cemetery is a ways off. The road that leads to it, paved with river stones, snakes between the houses and then, turning abruptly, climbs up the side of the hill, where the final resting places of the people of Berd keep multiplying, crowded against each other with their low fences. It's as if the people are trying to outdo each other in dying. It seems that only yesterday Razmik's grave was the one at the very end, but now you have to make your way past three rows just to get to it. Metaksia had picked a spot for him with plenty of room and plenty of open sky. She asked them to put him on the right side, in the shadow of the weeping willow. When her time comes, they'll put her on the left side; she's already made arrangements and even paid Tsatur, the gravedigger. Tsatur tried to turn down her money, but she insisted: "Look at you, all skin and bones. What if death comes to take me in the dead of winter, during the deep freeze? Where will you get the strength to dig up the frozen soil? This way, you'll pour yourself a nice bowl of hot bean soup, top it with some pork rinds, chase it down with a shot of cornelian cherry vodka . . . You'll enjoy it, and I will enjoy it too – it will be like I treated you to a meal!" Tsatur took the money, but when spring came, he showed up at Metaksia's doorstep and dug up her garden.

"What, can't bear to be separated from your shovel?" she joked.

"Yes, I've grown attached to it." Tsatur gave her a lopsided smirk and leaned into the handle of the shovel with his shoulder.

He has been coming over for years now. In the spring, he digs up the garden; in the autumn, he helps her pick potatoes and corn. At first, Metaksia kept trying to talk him out of it, but eventually she gave up. If he insists on coming back, he must need to be doing it, she figures. To show her gratitude, she knits winter hats with huge pompoms for Tsatur's kids. He has three little ones, one younger than the next. In those brightly colored hats, they look like cheerful little gnomes.

The silence that hangs over the cemetery is so thick that not even the thrush's trilling song can break it. Metaksia tidies up the grave with great care: she washes the fence and wipes it dry, pulls out the weeds, waters the flowers. As she cleans the accumulated dust and water stains off the gravestone, the years of birth and death etched on it emerge in silent reproach. She holds her breath for longer than she has the strength to. Is it ever possible to reconcile with the young ones dying? Seventeen years of age, an entire lifetime still waiting to be lived.

When she finishes tidying up, she measures frankincense into the memorial lamp and gently strikes a match. While the morning breeze scatters the slightly sweet-smelling, dense smoke, Metaksia sits on a low bench and looks off beyond the horizon, her hands folded in her lap. There, far in the distance, beyond the hunchbacked hill, lies her husband's grave. There's

---

Narine Abgaryan is the author of a dozen books; her book To Go On Living, *from which this excerpt was taken, was translated by Margarit Ordukhanyan and Zara Torlone, and published by* Plough *in April 2025. Abgaryan divides her time between Armenia and Germany.*

no reaching it now; the wind won't even carry her voice there.

Who could have thought that the happiness allotted to her would turn out to be so short-lived! She grew up in a loving home, with two parents and three older brothers. She never dreamed of getting married; she had been unlucky with her appearance – big-nosed, with a lazy eye and a lipless mouth. Having reconciled herself to her solitary lot, she looked after her numerous nieces and nephews, whom she adored more than life itself. But right after turning forty, she surprised even herself by marrying Razmik's father. They crossed the border to live in his hometown, Omarbeyli, a small hamlet with five Armenian families to seventy Azerbaijani ones.

Razmik was thirteen – a challenging, prickly age – and his father had a hard time dealing with him. People in the village felt sorry for the child: Poor orphan, it's not bad enough that he's lost his mother, but his father didn't even wait long before getting married again. Who has ever heard of a step-mother loving her stepson? She'll have her own kids and start trying to get rid of this one as soon as possible. Metaksia didn't really pay much heed to what people said, but deep down she also feared that having her own child might push Razmik away. That's why she never had the resolve to get pregnant.

Four years later, she lost her husband. He died in the middle of the night from a heart attack; he shrieked in pain, arched his back, accidentally hitting her with his elbow, and fell silent.

No matter how much Metaksia implored him, Razmik wouldn't hear of moving to Armenia. "I'm not going anywhere. I have school – I'm graduating this year!" he protested. She gave in but made him promise that they would move to Armenia for him to attend college. Razmik finally caved, on the condition that she would move his parents' ashes to Berd. His request offended her in earnest: "How could you even think that I'd abandon them!" He put his arms around her and broke into tears. From that day on, he took to calling her "Second Mom," or Second for short. She jokingly started calling him First. And so they lived, counting off – First-Second, Second-First.

When the war came, people in villages along the border didn't worry too much about it – all the families had been friends for decades and regularly visited each other. The war was somewhere out there, in the distance, and they were convinced that it wouldn't touch them. God willing, Metaksia rejoined with the rest. That was why she didn't worry when she went to visit her mother, who had taken ill, on the other side of the border. All she did was cook extra food and ask the neighbor to take the laundry off the line when it had dried because Razmik would never have remembered to. Late at night, word reached her that things were restive in Omarbeyli – sounds of gunfire reached the village from the border, and some houses were on fire.

It took Metaksia two full days to make it back. The house stood intact and unharmed; only

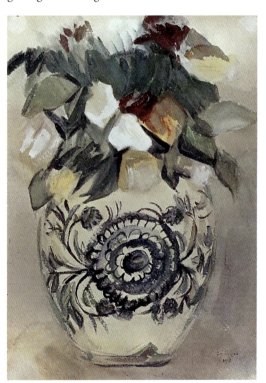

Martiros Sarian, *Vase*, 1913.

the gates were bent, as if from a heavy impact. Metaksia ran her fingers over the dent, feeling the roughness of mangled steel in bewilderment. The sheets, stiff from baking in the sun, hung from the laundry lines. It was so quiet inside the house that she could hear the beating of her own heart. Razmik wasn't inside. She eventually found him in the backyard, covered with some dirt and gardening tools that were haphazardly tossed over his body. Metaksia wiped the soil from his face and gathered it into her palms. Without pausing to think about what she was doing, she ate a handful of it, choking in horror and pain, and then poured the rest of it inside her blouse. She lit the stove and warmed up some water. From the cellar, she dragged up the huge basin that she normally used for soaking wool. She carefully laid Razmik inside it. She washed him gently, with bated breath, as if afraid to wake him up. Having realized that she had never once seen him naked before, she started whispering, to overcome her sudden feeling of embarrassment: "You are so well built, my boy, look at that beautiful body of yours. How handsome every part of you is, built for life, for joy, for happiness. If not for this wound in your belly . . . But I'll tie that up so that it doesn't ruin your beauty. I'll dress you in the suit we got for your graduation. I'll brush your unruly hair back – you never let me touch it, you just twisted your head and made annoyed faces, let me go, you said, it's fine as it is! You have such a big, bright forehead, and you wanted to keep it covered . . ."

She had to give up on the idea of putting on his shoes because she couldn't squeeze them on over his crushed feet. "Even killing can be done without inflicting unnecessary pain. Why the torture?" whispered Metaksia, as she wrapped Razmik's feet with towels. Then she dragged a cart out of the shed, lined it with a soft blanket, carefully placed Razmik in it, and rolled him out of their yard. The neighboring homes saw her off in hollow silence. Metaksia never even deigned to give them

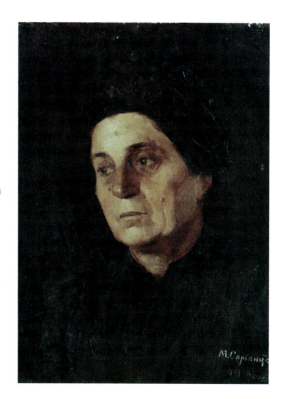

a parting glance. You say goodbye when you have something to say. She had nothing to say to them.

A gust of wind carried the sharp smell of pines and the distant voice of the awakening river. The sun painted the entire sky gold the moment it peeked from behind Maiden's Cliff.

Metaksia rose with a sigh, closed the lamp, and put it back into its special nook. She laid a slice of homemade bread at the head of the gravestone for the heavenly angels. She said goodbye, asked him not to worry and not to miss her too much, promising – Razmik-jan, I'll be back again next week. She left, having carefully shut the wicket gate behind her.

Berd was rising with the laughter of the children, with the coughing of the men, with the hushed voices of the women. Metaksia was walking down the slope, taking in the morning's breath. She had to hurry – the liturgy for the dead was about to begin. Needless to say, the dead have no use for it. The living, though, really need it. ✿

Martiros Sarian, *Portrait of Mother*, 1898.

Tights

In February, Mayinants Tsatur turned exactly as old as his father had been when he left for war. Tsatur still remembered how his mother, her arms wrapped around his father's neck, shook her head and begged him, in a voice gone hoarse from crying, "Please don't leave, I won't let you go!" Her bare feet dangled in the air. She was short of stature, with her head barely reaching her husband's shoulder, thin, almost translucent, light as a feather. For her delicate beauty, Arusiak had earned the nickname Doll. Everyone marveled at how a simple village woman could possess so much grace. She toiled in the fields and washed her linens in the river, but nonetheless resembled a porcelain figurine: delicate, slender, outlandish.

Tsatur was all of fourteen then, and he stood, pressing his weeping sisters to himself and summoning all of his strength to not break into tears himself. His father caught his eyes and mouthed to him: "Take her away." Tsatur gently took hold of his mother by her armpits and pulled her toward him. He expected her to resist, but she loosened her grip and went limp on his chest.

"Look after the girls," his father said curtly, and walked out without waiting for him to respond. That's how Tsatur remembered him: standing in the doorway, stooping a little – even though he knew that his head did not reach the top of the door frame, he still bent it slightly when he walked out the door. It was as if he shrank a little every time he left home.

Tsatur couldn't recognize his father in old photos: a large, prematurely gray-haired and incongruously happy man with sloping shoulders and eyes narrowed into tiny slits by laughter. The premature grayness turned out to be hereditary – Tsatur started going gray when he was still in high school and didn't have a single dark hair remaining in his mane by the time he turned thirty. His mother insisted that he looked just like his father; he didn't see the resemblance but didn't argue with her. Not that the resemblance brought her much comfort, but at least it made it easier for her to come to terms with her loss.

In late February, Tsatur turned thirty-three. His sisters came to visit, with their husbands and kids. Everyone stayed up late, reminiscing about childhood. Nobody brought up their father: they all preferred to think about him in private. The guests stayed until close to midnight. The kids were all nodding off by the warm wood-burning stove – bellies full, sleepy, having played their hearts out. While the sisters were saying their goodbyes, Tsatur's wife, Agnessa, handed out small presents: homemade necklaces for the girls, handmade *gulpa*[1] for the boys. The kids all kissed her hands, and only the youngest girl grabbed on to her and pulled her down toward her; her brother chastened her – Have you forgotten that it's hard for her? Tsatur picked up the little girl and brought her face to his wife's. She laughed and kissed the little girl on the nose. Their own children stood in a row, one younger than the next: a boy of five, another boy of four, and a two-and-a-half-year-old girl. Agnessa had always wanted a girl and finally got her wish.

They went to bed long after midnight: first they put the kids to sleep, then she did the dishes while he mopped the floors; she wouldn't have managed – it was hard for her to bend down, and she was exhausted after spending the entire day on her feet. "On her feet," Tsatur thought bitterly.

Agnessa, sensing his mood, asked, without turning away from the sink, "What are you thinking about?"

"About how hard things have gotten for you. Mom used to help, but now . . ." He stopped mid-sentence. She shrugged – this is not hard! He nodded in agreement. True, this is not hard.

Tsatur has been burying the people of Berd for seventeen years, ever since the day his father's remains were returned to them. That's when he went to the cemetery and asked Mehrab, the gravedigger, to teach him how to dig a proper grave.

1. Hand-knit woolen socks.

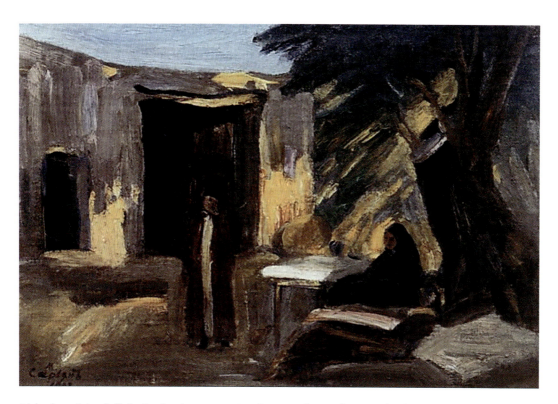

Mehrab explained all the intricacies concerning the depth and width of a grave, the properties of the soil and the groundwater. He explained where the head should be and drew a rectangle on the ground with the blade of his shovel. Tsatur handled the rest with his own two hands. While his mother and sisters were at home mourning his father, Tsatur readied his grave. After the funeral, he stayed to work at the cemetery, first as an apprentice to Mehrab, then, after his death, as the gravedigger. And so he lived, ferrying people between this world and the next. He selflessly dedicated himself to raising his sisters, making sure that first the older and then the younger finished school and got married. His mother fretted that he never got married, but he always dismissed her concerns: "Later, later. What talk can there be of marriage now, with so much grief around us?"

One time, he was asked to dig two child-sized graves. At the funeral, only one of the caskets was open. He assumed that the second child must have been maimed beyond recognition by an explosion, but somebody told him that the second casket contained a woman's legs. The family had been sheltering from a bombing in a cellar. It was cold out, and they didn't have time to get properly dressed – they had rushed out of the house in nothing but their sleepwear. The mother fretted that the girl might catch a cold and kept berating herself – if only I had grabbed warm tights for her, if only I had grabbed some tights. During a lull between explosions, she darted out to grab warm clothes, and her daughter chased after her. The child was killed by an explosion, and the mother had both of her legs blown off.

"She's alive, then?" asked Tsatur.

"You call that living?" came the retort.

He first saw Agnessa a few months later. She was sitting on the veranda of her father's house sorting peas. Her hair was cut short and tucked behind her ears, revealing a tiny pink scar on her left cheek, just below the cheekbone. Rumor had it that the scar was the handiwork of her former husband who never forgave her for the death of

Martiros Sarian, *Evening in the Garden*, 1903.

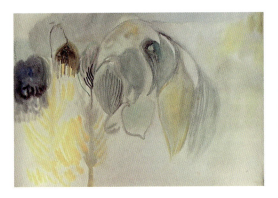

their child. Tsatur was stunned by the deathly pallor of her fingers and by how, even when she was finished with her task, she kept moving them, as if sorting the air. He watched her, unnoticed, for a while and then couldn't help asking, "Why do you keep moving your fingers?"

"It distracts me from my thoughts," she answered artlessly.

Her mother brought out steaming coffee in a *jezve*;[2] she didn't drink it herself but offered to read the grounds. The coffee patterns on the sides of the cup weren't promising: they portended disappointment, gossip, and worries. "I know what those worries are," said her mother plaintively, setting her cup aside, "I can't find prosthetic legs for her. I've been to town three times already, but no luck. She needs to learn to walk again!" She sighed and added bitterly, "My poor child." Agnessa leaned in and pressed her face to her mother's cheek. She didn't kiss her but just sat like that, her lips pressed against her mother's face, and there was so much tenderness and guilelessness in that gesture that Tsatur's heart felt a pinch.

"I'm going to town tomorrow anyway. Why don't you give me the clinic's address?" he said with a cough. And, in order to dispel any doubts, he added, hurriedly, "I have to go for work. I've got to buy a couple of tools."

He used the same pretext to explain his sudden trip to his own mother. Arusiak asked no questions, she just sighed.

Prosthetics were in high demand during the war, so civilian orders were constantly delayed. Nevertheless, Tsatur, after raising a considerable row at the clinic, managed to procure them. He ended up buying two bus tickets for his return trip; the prosthetic legs turned out to be so bulky that he couldn't just carry them in his arms, and he was afraid to put them in the luggage compartment – what if they got damaged? He traveled the entire way back with his arm over them in the seat next to his to keep them from sliding off.

Together, they learned how to do everything anew: how to walk, how to smile, how to breathe. Tsatur proposed with the arrival of spring. She asked him for some time to consider and accepted his proposal reluctantly, after much hesitation. There was no wedding – what revelry could there be amid so much grief? Agnessa dreamed of having a girl, but they had two boys back to back. The doctors, worried about her fragile health, recommended that she wait before having a third, but she didn't heed their advice and finally had a girl. She named her after her dead daughter because she firmly believed that if the name lived on, so did its bearer. Tsatur didn't try to talk his wife out of it even though he wasn't particularly thrilled with the idea of having his daughter named after a dead child. He never mentioned it – what was the point of discussing things that couldn't be changed? Agnessa loved her children more than life itself and always gave them everything they wanted. She fussed over them; she feared, to the point of panic, that they might catch a cold, and so, not sparing any expenses, bought them piles of winter clothes, to make sure they had spares and things to grow into: sweaters, jackets, warm boots, mittens, and scarves. The only thing she never bought were tights. So in the winter her kids waddled around like clumsy goslings, each wearing two pairs of woolen pants. And the funny hats with pompoms made for them by Ginamants Metaksia. ❈

2. A small pot with a long handle used for making coffee in Turkey, Armenia, and the Balkans.

Martiros Sarian, *Flowering Branch*, 1903.

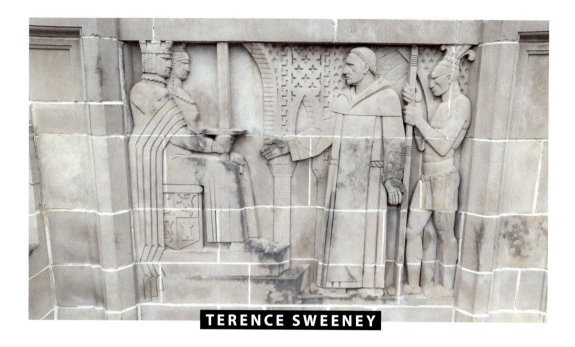

The Repentance of Bartolomé de las Casas

A slaveholding colonizer becomes a defender of the Indigenous.

TERENCE SWEENEY

A YOUNG PRIEST AT HIS DESK, slapping away the persistent flies, turns the pages of scripture, troubled by many things. He is not just any priest but a proud member of the las Casas family – a family close to Christopher Columbus – and resides in Hispaniola, one of the first Caribbean islands taken by the Spanish. He says Mass when he must but spends much of his time managing his *encomienda*, a plantation with a set number of Indigenous assigned as his slaves.

The priest is troubled by two recent experiences. He has just returned from serving as a chaplain during the conquest of Cuba. There he witnessed brutality, the likes of which he had never seen before. One story a Franciscan fellow chaplain told him stuck with him. Kneeling beside a dying chieftain, the Franciscan urged him to become Christian before he died so he could go to heaven. The chieftain asked if there were Christians in heaven. Upon being told yes, he shook his head; he "would rather go down to hell so he would not be where the Christians were, such cruel people."

The young priest was also anguished by the fiery words of Antonio de Montesinos, a Dominican friar who had, upon arriving in Hispaniola, demanded not just that the Spanish treat their

Lee Lawrie, *Las Casas Pleads for the Indian*, Indiana limestone relief, ca. 1922.

vestments, bread, and wine used at Mass – in short, everything that he as a priest offered to God – was literally stolen from the poor. These words of scripture cried out to him that his actions were worse than killing a son before his father's eyes. Who could continue, knowing that he had no right to any of this land, knowing that he was guilty of murder in God's eyes? And so, the young priest gave up his plantation, gave up being a well-off, complacent, slave-owning priest, and launched into a fifty-year campaign to defend the rights of the Indigenous to their land and freedom. He did this to follow the way of the Gospels and to share that way with others.

slaves well but that they *free them all*. "By what right or justice do you hold these Indians in such cruel and horrible slavery?" he proclaimed. "By what right do you wage such detestable wars on these people?" The young priest did not know by what right he blessed the Spanish conquerors of Cuba or sat in his study while enslaved Indigenous harvested sugar cane for him. There was no right he could think of to justify such things, nor could he square them with the gospel.

Turning the pages of his Bible to the Apocrypha, he settled on Ecclesiasticus, or Sirach. Saint Paul had his road to Damascus, where a light from heaven knocked him to the ground and he heard Christ calling to him, "Saul, Saul, why do you persecute me?" (Acts 9). Augustine heard "*tolle lege*" (take up and read) and took up and read that he must "put on Christ" (Rom. 12:4). In Ecclesiasticus, Bartolomé de las Casas found a passage that charged his heart: "Offering sacrifice from the property of the poor is as bad as slaughtering a son before his father's eyes" (34:20).

The land his chapel was on, and the offerings made by conquistadors that paid for the

THERE ARE FEW PEOPLE in history who have been as dynamic, impassioned, or active as Bartolomé de las Casas, who would go on to become Bishop of Chiapas, Mexico. He petitioned kings, governors, and popes. He argued with Renaissance scholars, spoke with Indigenous resistance fighters in the mountains, inspired young friars to join his work in the Americas, and endlessly enraged conquistadors. Abandoning his wealth, he took the poor habit of a Dominican friar and steeped himself in the thought of Thomas Aquinas, Augustine, and the scriptures.

He was not an easy man. Prone to exaggeration, he often inflated the numbers of Indigenous killed by the Spaniards. His outrage boiled over in an endless stream of polemics, but also found its way into his anthropological works, histories of the Spanish in the Americas, philosophical arguments, and guides for confessors. He crisscrossed the Atlantic multiple times, traveled to Mexico City, Cuba, and Hispaniola, and attempted to start a cooperative community for Spanish and Indigenous farmers in Venezuela. Kings wrote laws inspired by his writing, and the pope issued decrees based on his ideas.

Terence Sweeney is an assistant teaching professor in the Honors Program and Humanities Department at Villanova University.

A letter written by Bartolomé de las Casas.

None of this activity can be understood outside of the context of conversion. His life was deeply entwined with the realities of Spanish imperialism and thus he was often clearly in the wrong. But what made him unique was that he saw his own and his nation's wrongness and committed his life to repenting of sinful actions, changing the way he and Spain acted, and seeking to repair some of the damage caused by his and Spain's actions.

Las Casas was not a man without flaws. By the standards of many today, he was insufficiently critical of colonialism. Many now consider any attempt to convert the Indigenous to Christianity "religious colonialism." He was also an early advocate of enslaving Africans and bringing them to the New World. Some modern critics have held him responsible for the enslavement of thousands of Africans. They cite his 1516 request to King Charles V to send black slaves from Spain to replace Indigenous ones, which may have influenced Charles V's decision to approve the transport of four thousand African slaves to Jamaica in 1518. Others argue that the transatlantic slave trade was already underway and that las Casas's suggestions had little effect.

What is clear is that here again he later converted, writing, "I soon repented and judged myself guilty of ignorance. I came to realize that black slavery was as unjust as Indian slavery." Three centuries before the Emancipation Proclamation in the United States, las Casas demanded the end of African slavery in the Americas.

Thus, las Casas was a colonist who questioned colonization, a slave owner who questioned slave ownership, a coercive evangelizer who renounced coercion. He was a man of repentance who called upon his fellow Christians to repent. Seeing his own wrongdoing, he pointed out the wrongdoing of others. Knowing he had chosen the wrong path, he demanded that Christians take up the right path. He was prodigious, tireless, polemical, repentant, obsessed. As a critic of his wrote at the time, "He is a candle that sets everything afire wherever he goes."

L<small>AS</small> C<small>ASAS INSISTED</small> that Christian ethics had to be grounded in the gospel. He meant this in two senses. The first is that the preaching and witness of Christ is to be our only norm: to know how we are to be and act, we must always look to Christ's behavior and imitate him who teaches not just by words but by deeds. No doubt las Casas also drew on natural law, virtue ethics, and canon law, but the norm for these must always be Christ, because "what Christ did is law to us." If our natural law traditions run contrary to this incarnate, eternal law, then our interpretation of natural law needs to be changed or jettisoned.

Further, the gospel is *good news* – it is proclamatory. And the way we ought to proclaim it is with our lives; this should be the guiding principle for how we structure our entire lives. We must always ask ourselves, "What will these people think of Christ when they see us?" Las Casas learned this from the story of the dying chieftain who could not receive the good news as good because of the actions of its messengers. Not only must we imitate Christ, but we must do so publicly. The fundamental question is: Does my life attract others to Christ? There is, las Casas writes, "one way only, of teaching a living faith, to everyone, everywhere, always, set by Divine Providence; the way that wins the mind with reasons, that wins the will with gentleness, with invitation." Only if we live this way will the gospel be received as good news.

This understanding of mission led las Casas to champion universal human dignity. "All humanity is one" for las Casas because Christ set forth only one method for evangelizing: "Christ commanded: 'Go everywhere, teach everyone.' No one, no place is privileged. We are not to discriminate between places or persons." There can be no place for racism, coercion, or unjust treatment of anyone, because everyone is a recipient of the good news. When Christians use coercion of any kind, they make the good news bad news. "Who would want the gospel preached to him in such a fashion?" We must shape each moment of each day of our lives so that, through word and deed, people encounter in us a proclamation of the gospel.

The question of "by what right," for las Casas, is answered in the proclamation of the gospel according to the norm that is Christ. "Not by war. Not by force of arms. By the taste of peace. By an atmosphere of charity, by the works of kindness, of mercy, of modesty." The gospel means I have no right to war, injustice, exploitation, or harshness. I only have the right to offer freely what has been offered to me: faith, hope, and love. The question of what is right is thus determined by the good news as a *gift,* which must be offered "with gentleness." In being shaped by the gospel, I lose the false right to take; I gain the real right to give. Where the young las Casas took an *encomienda,* took slaves, and took part in colonizing, a deeper encounter with the gospel led him to *give* his whole life.

If the life of a Christian is always to imitate Christ, we live that life most especially in our care for the poor and suffering because, as las Casas says, "they are our brothers, redeemed by Christ's most precious blood." Christ's redemptive offering of his blood made humanity one family. Now no one is not my kin, no one is outside the order of my loves. But the oppressed need to come first because "God has a special memory for the smallest and the most forgotten." God holds the colonized, the enslaved, the unborn, the refugee, the poor, the neglected old and ill in his memory and requires that we too keep them close. The good news is primarily for them.

What is right, las Casas says, must be shaped by the reality of the situation. And what was the situation? That a son was being murdered before the eyes of his father. For las Casas, Ecclesiasticus 34:20 was no abstraction. It was the image of the Son of God on the cross, murdered by us. It was also what he found in the New World: "Jesus Christ, our God, scourged and afflicted and beaten and crucified not once but thousands of times." The reality is that those we oppress or neglect *are Christ and him crucified*. To worship rightly thus is not only to cease to oppress but to stand in solidarity with Christ crucified in the oppressed.

A**N OLD PRIEST AT HIS DESK** takes up his pen as he has so many times before. He writes to the pope to tell him that the Indigenous are "capable of understanding the gospel and eternal life." The old bishop considers the many successes and failures in his life. He has helped end slavery in Mexico and inspired countless friars to bring the gospel peacefully to the New World. But also there on his desk he has a letter from Indigenous leaders begging him to represent their cause in the Spanish court. His attempts to stop the destruction of Indigenous peoples have mostly been ignored. Spanish seminaries have refused his call to accept Indigenous men into formation for the priesthood. The African slave trade has grown while the Indigenous population of the Caribbean islands has collapsed.

Does he despair? No, he takes pen to paper once again. The gospel does not promise him success. In a world that rejects the refugee, aborts the young, euthanizes the old, exploits the labor of the poor, and rejects the gospel, we too are not promised success. What we are given instead is a deeper story of "goodness going out and goodness coming back." Las Casas calls us to commit to being a part of that goodness, to join him in following goodness incarnate in Christ, in defending everyone's right to hearing the gospel with love, and in offering worship in solidarity with Christ, the divine Son, and all the crucified sons and daughters of the Father.